Advice for the Novice Investigator

Advice for the Novice Investigator
Examples Taken from Movement Sciences

Nick Stergiou

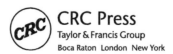

CRC Press
Taylor & Francis Group
Boca Raton London New York

CRC Press is an imprint of the
Taylor & Francis Group, an **informa** business

CRC Press
Taylor & Francis Group
6000 Broken Sound Parkway NW, Suite 300
Boca Raton, FL 33487-2742

Library of Congress Cataloging-in-Publication Data

Names: Stergiou, Nicholas, author.
Title: Advice for the novice investigator : examples taken from movement
sciences / by Nick Stergiou.
Description: Boca Raton : Taylor & Francis, a CRC title, part of the Taylor &
Francis imprint, a member of the Taylor & Francis Group, the academic
division of T&F Informa, plc, 2019. | Includes bibliographical references.
Identifiers: LCCN 2019017959 | ISBN 9781138626188 (hardback : acid-free
paper) |
ISBN 9781315229690 (e-book)
Subjects: LCSH: Science—Vocational guidance.
Classification: LCC Q147 .S73 2019 | DDC 502.3—dc23
LC record available at https://lccn.loc.gov/2019017959

Visit the Taylor & Francis Web site at
http://www.taylorandfrancis.com

and the CRC Press Web site at
http://www.crcpress.com

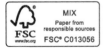

Printed and bound in Great Britain by
TJ International Ltd, Padstow, Cornwall

This book is dedicated to all my students, past, present, and future.

Contents

Preface

When you start on your journey to Ithaca, then pray
that the road is long,
full of adventure, full of knowledge. Do not fear the
Lestrygonians
and the Cyclopes and the angry Poseidon...
Always keep Ithaca fixed in your mind. To arrive
there is your ultimate goal

> *From the poem* Ithaca *of Konstantinos*
> *Kavafis (1863–1933) who was an Egyptiot*
> *Greek poet, journalist, and civil servant.*

Success in science is not easy. A scientist has to face many adversities exactly like Odysseus, the hero of Homer's epic poem *The Odyssey*, on his trip to Ithaca. The road to success will be laid with many Lestrygonians and Cyclopes. The sea will be sparingly calm, and you may feel that Poseidon is always angry with you. Ramon Y. Cajal, the father of modern neurobiology, captured this sense as he wrote in his book entitled *Advice to a Young Investigator* 100 years ago: "more than once I was hopelessly discouraged about my ability to pursue science." This is one of the reasons that he wrote a book to help young scientists, providing them with advice on how to overcome adversities and arrive at their scientific Ithaca. However, as someone peruses his book can also see that Cajal did have another very strong motivation, his love towards his students and young apprentices.

I believe this is what I have in common with the great Cajal. Certainly, I do not have a Nobel Prize as he did, and I made many more mistakes in my scientific career. When I reflect back on more than 20 years of being a professor and administrator and 11 more as an undergraduate and graduate student, I see plenty of mistakes. However, I love my students and apprentices very much. Maybe the fact that I do not have my own children is one reason I channel all my love towards them. This is why, even from the beginning of my career, I have spent my time with immense gladness in advising, mentoring, and teaching young people how to avoid all the mistakes that I have made. This is why, almost 10 years ago, I started a course in my department where I teach young scientists how to avoid the same mistakes I made. The topics in this course range from how to handle ethical situations, how to write grants and manuscripts, how to present, and many others. I have a great number of people attending my course, from young faculty to senior undergraduates. Their praise of my sincerity for this purpose has been a continuous motivation. They have also encouraged me to publish this knowledge so many others can benefit. I have also received such encouragement from colleagues in other universities who have similar noble aspirations towards their young scientists but lack a comprehensive textbook on the subject matter.

This is why I finally decided to grant these requests and write such a book. The organization of our book is as follows: In the first chapter, I discuss how a scientist can become an effective detective and maximize enjoyment in this profession. This is accomplished by presenting, in detail, an article published in 1964 by John Rader Platt titled "Strong inference." In the second chapter, I provide a comprehensive approach, along with numerous examples and tips, on how to get your grant proposals funded. In addition, I provide tips on organizing and producing a successful research plan with novel ideas, the foundation for good grantsmanship. In the third chapter, I teach you how to write successful grant proposals. Emphasis is given to writing grants for the National Institutes of Health (NIH). As one of my grant writing mentors, Dr. Jeff French once said, "if you know how to write grants for the NIH, you can write for any agency and funding source."

One of the most fundamental aspects of academic life is writing scientific manuscripts. Thus, in the fourth chapter, I aim to assist novice investigators in writing scientific manuscripts and identifying critical writing mistakes. These skills are also important for anyone who wishes to write in science. In the fifth chapter, I focus on responsible conduct in research, including topics related to authorship, supervisory and mentoring relationships, and other scientific tasks.

In the sixth chapter, I discuss a number of important skills regarding time and laboratory management and organization that are needed in order to become a successful scientist and academician. However, many of these skills, and my corresponding advice, also apply to employment in industry and life, more generally. For example, knowing how to effectively manage your time is an issue that stresses almost everybody in our modern societies. I continue in the same realm with the seventh chapter but discuss other skills that range the spectrum from teaching a class to negotiating a deal. I finish the book with the eighth chapter where I provide a variety of motivational tools for young investigators.

These tools are advices, quotes, and even selected passages from short biographies such as obituaries, from great scientists demonstrating how they accomplished such greatness. They also provide invaluable information on these scientists' general characteristics. Such information can guide the young investigators in shaping their own character.

For any fellow teachers that would like to use this book for similar courses or want to create a course based on the material presented here, I have tried to help them by developing some slides that accompany each chapter. These slides are by no means complete as they do not cover this book word by word. However, I believe that they are a good starting point.

Examples are aplenty throughout the book. However, a disclaimer needs to be made. These examples are derived mostly from my own scientific area which is movement science, in general. This disclaimer is made because the book may have a wider appeal. However, my limits are obvious. Another disclaimer is that the advice that I provide comes with all humility attached to it, as I have declared that I have made every mistake possible. Hopefully, the young investigators that read this book will have a much safer trip than me and more favorable winds in their sails as they travel towards their Ithaca.

Another disclaimer that needs to be made is regarding the significant financial support that I have received over the years by several agencies. The NIH, NASA, U.S. Department of Education, National Science Foundation, Department of Veterans Affairs, Nebraska Research Initiative, and many others have consistently provided funds for my work and allowed me to progress with financial stability over the years. I am particularly grateful to the NIH and National Institute of General Medical Sciences for a COBRE P20GM109090 grant that I have recently received that supported the writing of this book the past year.

Lastly, I acknowledge that during my life I have faced, more than once, adversity and disappointment. Such times have also been aplenty in my career and not only in the development, of this book but also in the investigation of a novel area of research that is different from traditional approaches. In these times, there is one certainty that solace is needed around you to overcome even the highest of obstacles. This is why I am eternally grateful to my parents, Jesus and Vaya, my brother, Dimitris and his family, my mentors, Dr. Barry Bates, Dr. Janet Dufek, and Dr. Jody Jensen, my American parents, Ruth and Bill Scott and the entire Scott family, my friends and collaborators, and particularly my students for their love, support, and constant encouragement. In particular, I am grateful to my doctoral student, Dr. Jenny Kent, and my good friend, Dr. Aaron Likens, who read and provided comments for every single chapter of this book.

Author

Dr. Nick Stergiou is the Distinguished Community Research chair in Biomechanics and professor as well as the director of the Biomechanics Research Building and the Center for Research in Human Movement Variability at the University of Nebraska at Omaha where his primary appointment is. Recently, he was also appointed as the assistant dean of the Division of Biomechanics and Research Development. He is the founding chair of the first ever academic Department of Biomechanics that graduates students with a BS in Biomechanics. His secondary appointment is as a professor of the Department of Environmental, Agricultural, and Occupational Health of the College of Public Health at the University of Nebraska Medical Center. His research focuses on understanding variability inherent in human movement, and he is an international authority in the study of nonlinear dynamics. He has been inducted to the National Academy of Kinesiology and as a fellow to the American Institute for Medical and Biological Engineering. Dr. Stergiou's research spans from infant development to older adult fallers and has impacted training techniques of surgeons and treatment and rehabilitation of pathologies, such as peripheral arterial disease. He has received more than $30 million in personal funding from NIH, NASA, NSF, the NIDRR/U.S. Department of Education, and many other agencies and foundations. He has received the largest grant in the history of his university, a NIH P20 grant that was worth $10.1 million. This grant allowed him to develop the Center for Research in Human Movement Variability. He has also several inventions and has procured a private donation of $6 million to build the 23,000-square-foot Biomechanics Research Building that has opened in August 2013. This is the first building dedicated to biomechanics research in the world. It is also the first building on his campus exclusively dedicated to research. Recently, he has procured $11.6 million to build a 30,000-square-foot expansion to this building.

chapter one

Strong inference

It would have a salutary effect on our attitudes if for twenty-four hours we could cross out the words "science" and "scientist" whenever they appear, and out in their place the words "man reasoning." Even in the mathematical sciences, like physics, it is the reasoning that comes first, the equations second; and the equations will not save the theory if the reasoning is wrong. It cannot be said too often that science is not mathematics, but reasoning; not equipment, but inquiry.

—John Rader Platt (1918–1992)

1.1 Introduction

To be a scientist is extremely enjoyable. I tell this to everybody. However, many people listen to me in great disbelief. How can someone enjoy spending hours and days and years closed inside a laboratory? How can someone live as an ascetic? There are many reasons that I will mention in several places of this book, but the main one is the enjoyment that comes from following a chain of reasoning and trying to solve a mystery. You place yourself in the middle of a Sir Conan Doyle book as a modern-day Sherlock Holmes; you are a detective that is trying to solve intriguing puzzles. I remember quite vividly some of my students running to my office to celebrate an exciting new finding in the laboratory. What gives them such a pleasure, such a thrill? Discovery!

Therefore, in this first chapter, I would like to present how a scientist can become an effective detective and maximize enjoyment in this profession. This is accomplished by presenting in detail an article published in 1964 by John Rader Platt titled "Strong inference" (Platt, 1964). This is an article that I ask all my students to read for the first day of classes. I consider it fundamental for scientists and the most important article that I have ever read. I am also aware that the article has significant following across several disciplines.

1.2 Strong inference: The Definition

John Rader Platt (1918–1992) was an American biophysicist and professor at the University of Chicago. In 1964, he published an article in *Science* titled "Strong inference." Platt defined strong inference as an excellent model of scientific inquiry that emphasizes the need for alternative hypotheses. In this fashion, you do not use a single hypothesis, and thus, you avoid confirmation bias. Confirmation bias is the inclination to search and interpret data in a way that corroborates preexisting hypotheses. It is also a systematic error of inductive reasoning and contributes to the preservation of hypotheses even in the face of contrary evidence. In my career, I have seen such a preservation of hypotheses and theoretical perspectives several times.

Platt mentioned in his article that certain fields, such as molecular biology, follow tightly strong inference, and as a result, they have tremendous results and significant progress. I believe that it is important for every scientist to always reflect on his/her own discipline and consider if this is also the case. Do you see significant advancements? Do you see discoveries that jump out from the front pages of newspapers and are shared on social media? If not, why not? Is it because strong inference is not followed? Strong inference, as a method of reasoning and analytical thinking, uses the elimination of alternative hypotheses to focus thinking and devise a logical stream of experiments. Such an engagement in the scientific process leads to very quick and powerful conclusions. Platt described the four steps of strong inference (Table 1.1) but also mentioned that this is not something new as it goes back to Francis Bacon (1561–1626). Interestingly, every scientist is aware of this process. However, it is not used systematically and is not part of the daily routine. Instead, many scientists simply conduct another survey, another more detailed study, another descriptive study. What we really need is for scientists to consider alternative hypotheses, develop and execute crucial experiments, and have their laboratory notebooks full of "logical trees" of sequential experiments and results.

Table 1.1 The four steps of strong inference

---

1. Devising alternative hypotheses;
2. Devising a crucial experiment (or several of them), with alternative possible outcomes, each of which will, as nearly as possible, exclude one or more of the hypotheses;
3. Carrying out the experiment so as to get a clean result;
4. Recycling the procedure, making sub hypotheses or sequential hypotheses to refine the possibilities that remain; and so on.

Source: Platt (1964, p. 347).

Among the four steps (Table 1.1), I believe that the most difficult is devising the crucial experiment. This is because it requires a lot of critical thinking and a great deal of patience. Often, a crucial experiment is extremely elegant and may not conform to other people's logical thinking. Continuous attendance to the world's literature assists in developing crucial experiments, as it allows the scientist to update the logical tree of experimental work in their laboratory notebooks. This needs to be done on a daily basis. Here are some hints to help you with this process:

1. As soon as you read a new result in the world's literature or it comes out from your laboratory, place it on the top of a page in your laboratory notebook to start a new logical tree or continue with the previous one that you constructed before.
2. Right underneath, write two or three alternative explanations or limitations or what you believe was done incorrectly.
3. Below that, write suggested experiments or studies that can practically eliminate these explanations.
4. Continue this process with discipline and the "logical tree" slowly grows.
5. Support this growth with discussions with colleagues and fellow scientists in journal clubs and in social meetings.

The above process can also be performed by an entire laboratory team. In the 1950s, several big laboratories around the world used big chalkboards to facilitate this process (Platt, 1964). For example, in the Laboratory of Molecular Biology in Cambridge, England, the chalkboards of the famous Francis Crick (who received the Nobel Prize for the DNA helix) were commonly found covered with logical trees. The laboratory team had a massive logical tree and would fit into it every new finding they gained from searching the literature in the library. They would state their hypotheses based on those results and eliminate them one by one as they were disproved. They were all working together on the logical tree. Maybe each one of them had his own logical tree, but they had a common one as well. A few years ago, when I went to Cambridge, I actually tried to find these chalkboards, hoping they had kept them. They had not. The only thing that was still around from those times was in the bar (the "Eagle") across the street, where there were pictures of James Watson and Francis Crick. The pictures were taken during the press conference that was held at that bar regarding the Nobel Prize for the DNA helix. Watson and Crick used the bar as a place to relax and discuss their "logical trees" while refreshing themselves with ale.

To better comprehend strong inference and the ensuing "logical tree" of sequential experiments and results, let us consider a few examples.

1.3   Examples of strong inference

1.3.1   Molecular biology

In 1953, Watson and Crick proposed that the DNA molecule is composed of two chains that coil around each other to form a double helix (Watson & Crick, 1953; Platt, 1964). Their model of DNA was based on a result from Franklin and Gosling (an X-ray diffraction image; Franklin & Gosling, 1953) and additional information that the DNA bases are paired. This proposition suggested a number of alternative hypotheses to design crucial experiments. One such alternative hypothesis was related to what happens with the DNA double helix during cell division, specifically if the two chains separate or if they stay together. Meselson and Stahl found that they separate. They used an elegant crucial experiment that was based on an ingenious isotope-density labeling technique (Meselson & Stahl, 1958). Another alternative hypothesis was related to the number of chains that exist on the DNA helix, specifically if they are two or three. Rich showed that it can have either (Rich, 1958). It is actually a worthwhile exercise to read papers from the molecular biology scientific giants of those times and observe how effectively these papers radiate strong inference, describing experiments that eliminate alternative hypotheses.

1.3.2   Motor control and development

Reflex hierarchical theory (RHT) of motor control and dynamical systems theory (DST) will be discussed in brief to examine if the research driven by these theoretical perspectives follows the guidelines of strong inference (Platt, 1964). These theories will be examined from a locomotion/developmental standpoint. RHT is based on two major concepts: (a) the central nervous system (CNS) is organized hierarchically with the lower structures controlled by higher nervous centers, and (b) a sensory input is needed for a motor output. RHT was developed from the pioneering work of Sherrington (1898, 1906). Originally, Sherrington developed the following hypothesis: locomotion is initiated from the CNS, where central pattern generators (CPGs) exist, and sensory feedback is not necessary. Experiments were then conducted to test the alternative hypothesis that sensory feedback from the periphery is necessary for locomotion. On performing a low thoracic transection of a cat's spinal cord, it was shown that the cat was still able to perform locomotor movements while suspended in the air. When a unilateral cut of the dorsal nerves was performed (thereby eliminating the sensory feedback on locomotion on one side of the body), it was found that the cat could not use the deafferented limb during locomotion. It was then hypothesized that the stereotypic motor responses occurring following sensory inputs are reflexes, and complex movements like locomotion are a chaining of many reflexes together

(Sherrington, 1898, 1906). Brown (1911) found that movements still persisted for a few minutes following a bilateral cut of the dorsal roots in cats, lending support to the alternative hypothesis that sensory inputs are necessary. Taub and Berman (1968) observed that cats will not use a limb when the dorsal roots are cut unilaterally but regain the use of this limb with a bilateral cut. This supported the original Sherrington hypothesis that locomotion is initiated from the CNS, where CPG exists, and sensory feedback is not necessary.

This initial work and evidence, in favor of the notion of CPG, led to a new question: since a CPG exists, where is it located? Shik et al. (1966) showed that locomotion can be produced by an electrical stimulation of the brain stem of a decerebrate cat. They concluded that higher nervous system centers control movement. They called this area the mesencephalic locomotor region. To test the alternative hypothesis that CPG is not located at the brain, Grillner (1973) extended the Sherrington experiments by giving descending stimulation to the mesencephalic locomotor region and by applying levodopa to the spinal cord. They found that walking was generated with low rates of repetitive stimulation, with trot and eventually gallop generated with even higher rates of repetitive stimulation. In addition, they found that despite cutting the spinal cord just above the hind limbs, the animal could still walk when supported on a treadmill. These results support the alternative hypothesis that the CPG is at the spinal cord and not higher at the CNS.

The next branch of the experimental tree was to investigate whether the CPG is located at the spinal cord or is even lower, that is, every leg has its own CPG or there is one CPG for all legs (Grillner, 1973). So, the same spinalized cat was placed on a split treadmill such that the two sides could move at two different speeds. Amazingly, the cat was able to accommodate the two different speeds. This showed the existence of independent pattern generators. However, besides the presence of locomotion, Grillner and colleagues found differences between spinalized and deafferented cats, such as the time between the midpoint of two repetitions of a muscle burst (Grillner & Zangger, 1979; Grillner & Rossignol, 1978). This led to the hypothesis that besides the CPG, the sensory input might also contribute to locomotion, which leads us back to the original Sherrington hypothesis. Experimental results showed that the position of the hip joint of the ipsilateral leg was a key factor in the initiation of the swing phase in locomotion. When extension of the hip was maximized, it was activating flexion, and when extension was blocked, the swing phase was inhibited. Thus, they concluded that sensory input was important for locomotion without refuting the existence of CPG.

The above experimental work was concentrated in animals. Therefore, the next step was to apply these ideas to human research. Forssberg (1985) observed that newborns (5–6 days old) were able to perform a step or a series of steps. However, these patterns disappeared after 2 months of age. The patterns then reappeared, first in crawling, and then in walking. Primitive reflexes in newborns were offered as an explanation for this behavioral pattern, and it was suggested that neural maturation is necessary to achieve locomotion. This neural maturation can be viewed as the evolution of a CPG that rewires the original or modifies it.

Based on the above, we observe that even though the presence of strong inference is evident, a tremendous amount of research effort was spent to identify the location of elements responsible for generation of locomotion, and little effort was spent in answering the originating, critical question: How are these elements coordinated to generate locomotion (Woollacott & Jensen, 1996; Smith & Thelen, 1994)? The same can be inferred from the modular or systems theory, where other biological structures such as the cerebellum (Keele et al., 1987) have been suggested as structures that could modulate locomotion. This may explain the existence of a number of theories in motor control. Platt (1964) actually uses biology as a good example to what might have happened in motor control. He stated,

> Biology with its vast informational detail and complexity, is a high information field, where years and decades can easily be wasted on the usual type of low information observations or experiments if one does not think carefully in advance about what the most important and conclusive experiments would be.

Furthermore, as Platt suggested (1964), one should always ask "what experiment could disprove the hypothesis." For instance, in the case of the disappearance of stepping reflex in infants and the explanation proposed by Forssberg (1985), the alternative hypothesis can be supported if an experiment can be conducted to show that the stepping reflex is intact. One such experiment is the placement of the infants in water (buoyancy decreases the leg's weight which due to development may have become too heavy for the pattern to be exhibited). If the infant can perform well-coordinated steps in water, the alternative hypothesis will be supported, and another explanation other than neuromaturation will be needed. When Thelen et al. (1984) performed the above experiment, they reported results in support of an alternate hypothesis to neuromaturation. Further experiments showed that when weights were placed on the infants' legs (simulating an increase in mass), the behavior was no longer exhibited. It was then hypothesized that motor output is not the product of one factor, like neuromaturation (Forssberg, 1985), but the result of an integration or self-organization of the external and internal constraints of the system. It was concluded that a systems integration perspective is needed to understand the motor behavior. Thelen (1986) also tested this approach by placing supported infants over a small, motorized treadmill.

She found that the infants showed immediate alternating stepping, similar to adultlike steps. Thelen concluded that the DST approach provides a dynamic flexibility of behavior that can explain discontinuities in motor skill development. To further test the self-organization notion, Thelen et al. (1987) placed 7-month-old infants on a split treadmill where each leg moved backward at a different rate. Amazingly, the infants were able to adjust their stepping pattern to maintain the half phase lag of an alternating gait. They concluded that the coordinated alternating stepping was not a result of either an intrinsic rhythm generator or the treadmill's speed alone, but it was the ability of the system's self-organization from its elements that produced the observed behavior. The above experimental work led to the final form of DST and has been described in detail by Thelen and Ulrich (1991).

1.3.3 Biomechanics and orthopedic surgery

Anterior cruciate ligament (ACL) injury is practically an epidemic in sports. Nowadays, everyone participates in sports, and that leads to more ACL injuries. ACL injury, even with a reconstruction, leads to osteoarthritis which eventually requires knee replacement. So why do we get osteoarthritis after an ACL injury, even when a reconstruction is performed? Is it because we still do not know how to perform a reconctruction properly? These are fundamental questions. The search for solutions raises several more questions along different possible avenues. Should I reconstruct the ACL using animal ligaments, which have very similar ligaments to humans? Should I design a nonbiological graft using 3D printing? What type of a graft should I use? What type of surgery should I perform? Most importantly, does an ACL reconstruction (the current standard of care) truly lead to restoration of function? A group of scientists and orthopedic surgeons worked together in Greece trying to address some of these questions. In their laboratory, they actually had a logical tree on a chalkboard that was similar to the one used by Crick and colleagues in Cambridge (see Section 1.3.1). They added all the results to that logical tree as they emerged. The senior orthopedic surgeon was always excited about the publication date because many scientists were asking about the newest experimental results. Science is pure enjoyment and, when done properly, gives you this amazing investigative feeling, like you are another Sherlock Holmes.

This group started with the following hypothesis: An ACL reconstruction will result in a patient being able to perform physical activities exactly as before. Then they thought of an experiment that can disprove this hypothesis. They developed a simple experiment where they compared individuals that had an ACL deficiency, an ACL reconstruction, and no ACL injury (matched healthy controls) during walking (Georgoulis et al., 2003). Similar to other results in the literature, they found mostly no differences, as normal movement patterns were maintained. However, in ACL-deficient individuals, there was an important finding; tibial transverse plane rotation was significantly different from that of healthy controls. This observation was not apparent after reconstruction. But, is it possible that walking was not the appropriate task to reveal biomechanical differences in the transverse plane in the reconstructed individuals? Because walking does not really have a strong rotational component, is the tibial rotation that was found to be significantly larger in ACL-deficient individuals really improved after an ACL reconstruction? Therefore, they investigated an activity with a strong rotational component, such as pivoting. They conducted an experiment where they compared individuals that had an ACL deficiency, an ACL reconstruction, and no ACL injury (matched healthy controls) performing physical activities with strong rotational components, for example, descending stairs and pivoting or jumping from a platform and pivoting (Ristanis et al., 2003, 2005, 2006). They found that excessive tibial rotation during such physical activities is not restored after an ACL reconstruction. This led them to the following question: Is it possible that the way that ACL reconstruction is performed is actually responsible for this result? If you use a different procedure, do you get better results? Therefore, they conducted an experiment in which they compared individuals that have had an ACL reconstruction with a hamstring graft with others that had this procedure performed using a patellar tendon graft (Chouliaras et al., 2007). They found no difference in terms of tibial rotation between the two grafts. This result creates other questions as well. Maybe there is a need to perform the procedure in a different way (Ristanis et al., 2009). Maybe there is a need to use a different rehabilitation approach besides the reconstruction (Giotis et al., 2011). Is tibial rotation actually a problem? Does the tibial rotation lead to mechanical deformities that result in future problems? Is osteoarthritis common in people with ACL deficiency because of tibial rotation? What is the mechanism that causes the osteoarthritis (Stergiou et al., 2007)? And your logical tree expands...

1.4   Additional thoughts on strong inference

A critical question that is raised at this point is, why is what has been described above in these three examples not performed all the time and by every scientist?

There are multiple reasons for this problem. One of them is that many scientists and even entire disciplines become too method oriented. Platt (1964) states,

> Beware of the man of one method or one instrument, either experimental or theoretical. He tends

> to become method-oriented rather than problem
> oriented. The method-oriented man is shack-
> led: the problem-oriented man is at least reaching
> freely toward what is most important. Strong infer-
> ence redirects a man to problem-orientation, but it
> requires him to be willing repeatedly to put aside
> his last methods and teach himself new ones.

I attended an American Society of Biomechanics meeting a few years ago
in Long Beach with my previous doctoral student. He was presenting a
study that challenged a well-known theoretical paradigm. His experiment was one of disproof. The room was absolutely packed. Next door
there was someone talking of yet another method of placing markers to
about ten people. Almost nobody was attending. People are "hungry" for
experiments that radiate strong inference, for good science, and not for
another descriptive study. Many times, we praise a "lifetime of study"
but truly what is really needed in every field is not a lifetime but maybe
a few months of systematic application of strong inference. One of the
most amazing things happens to you when you follow this investigative
approach. The next experiment becomes vivid. Usually, the phenomenon
is right there to grasp, but you can't always see it without this approach.

Another reason for the lack of application of strong inference is that
many scientists become too attached to their hypothesis and do not seek
its disproof. However, as Platt states, "a theory which cannot be mortally
endangered cannot be alive." A Physics professor of mine at the University
of Oregon, Dr. Russ Donnelly, also used to say that "99% of theories will
go to the garbage can. So, don't be too attached to them." I completely
agree with these statements, and I always emphasize them in my research
seminars. Do not get too attached to your theory, and keep your ego in
check at all times. I always advise the young scientists to give a name
to the garbage cans in their offices. Call it ego! I have a piece of paper
glued on mine that has "EGO" written on it. Always ask yourself what
experiment will disprove your theory. When you go to a scientific meeting, ask the same question to other scientists. It will certainly provoke
very interesting discussions.

On the other hand, being involved in science without a theory is similar to being lost in the middle of nowhere without a map. This is exactly
why you need strong inference and its systematic application – to know
where you are going in your scientific investigations. Therefore, if I am
going to propose a theory, I need to be able to propose experiments that
will disprove this theory. Otherwise, it is dogma. A good theory has two
characteristics. It must (a) describe a large group of observations and (b)
provide predictions about the results of future observations (Hawking,
1998). Practically, a theory gives meaning to facts, just as a blueprint

provides the structure that transforms stones into a house (Miller, 2002). If you have no theory or testable hypotheses, you just produce stones that lay around the yard!

1.5   *Strong inference – take-home messages*

- Develop your logical tree and a focused line of research using strong inference. Now, when you are still young, and I am talking about both graduate students and junior faculty members, you need to try and establish this as your foundation.
- Be problem oriented, not method oriented. Always ask "how I can disprove my theory?" or "what hypothesis will my experiment disprove?" This should be your first and main objective when creating a research question. Also ask "what is the next logical step, based on my current findings?" or "how does this finding relate to my logical tree?"
- With an intelligent employment of scientific theory, you can arrive at new insights and conclusions. If you are conducting random experiments without specific hypotheses and without strong inference, then you are not building a scientific house; you are not developing a logical tree. You are not a scientist.
- Devote at least half an hour a day to critical and analytical thinking. During this time, write and refine your logical tree, your alternative hypotheses, and your crucial experiments in your laboratory notebook. The famous mathematician Gauss used to say that "if others would but reflect on mathematical truths as deeply and continuously as I have, they would make my discoveries." And when Newton was asked how he made discoveries surpassing those of his predecessors, he replied, "by always thinking about them." Lastly, Goldberger used to say that "there are some problems you cannot solve in a million years unless you think about them for five minutes" (Bell, 1986).

References

Bell, E.T. (1986). *Men of Mathematics. A Touchtone Book*. New York: Simon & Schuster, Inc.

Brown, T.G. (1911). The intrinsic factors in the act of progression in the mammal. *Proceedings of the Royal Society, London*, 84, 308–319.

Chouliaras, V., Ristanis, C., Moraiti, C., Stergiou, N., Georgoulis, A.D. (2007). Effectiveness of reconstruction of the anterior cruciate ligament with qua- drupled hamstrings and bone-patellar tendon-bone autografts: an in vivo study comparing tibial internal-external rotation. *American Journal of Sports Medicine*, 35(2), 189–196.

Forssberg, H. (1985). Ontogeny of human locomotor control I. Infant stepping, supported locomotion and transition to independent locomotion. *Experimental Brain Research*, 57, 480–493.

Franklin, R.E., Gosling, R.G. (1953). Molecular configuration in sodium thymonucleate. *Nature*, 171(4356), 740–741.

Georgoulis, A.D., Papadonikolakis, A., Papageorgiou, C.D., Mitsou, A., Stergiou, N. (2003). Three-dimensional tibiofemoral kinematics of the anterior cruciate ligament-deficient and reconstructed knee during walking. *American Journal of Sports Medicine*, 31(1), 75–79.

Giotis, D., Tsiaras, V., Ristanis, S., Zampeli, F., Mitsionis, G., Stergiou, N., Georgoulis, A.D. (2011). Knee braces can decrease tibial rotation during pivoting that occurs in high demanding activities. *Knee Surgery Sports Traumatology and Arthroscopy*, 19(8), 1347–1354.

Grillner, S. (1973). Locomotion in the spinal cat. In R.B. Stein, K.G. Pearson, R.S. Smith, & J.B. Redford (Eds.), *Control of Posture and Locomotion* (pp. 515–535). New York: Plenum.

Grillner, S., Rossignol, S. (1978). On the initiation of the swing phase of locomotion in chronic spinal cats. *Brain Research*, 146, 269–277.

Grillner, S., Zangger, P. (1979). On the central generation of locomotion in the low spinal cat. *Experimental Brain Research*, 34, 241–261.

Hawking, S.W. (1998). *A Brief History of Time*. London: Bantam.

Keele, S.W., Ivry, R.I., Pokormy, R.A. (1987). Force control and its relationship to timing. *Journal of Motor Behavior*, 19, 96–144.

Meselson, M., Stahl, F. (1958). The replication of DNA in *E. coli*. *Proceedings of the National Academy of Sciences of the United States of America*, 44(7), 671–682.

Miller, P.H. (2002). *Theories of Developmental Psychology*. 4th Edition. New York: Worth Publishers.

Platt, J.R. (1964). Strong inference. Certain systematic methods of scientific thinking may produce much more rapid progress than others. *Science*, 146(3642), 347–353.

Rich, A. (1958). Formation of two- and three-stranded helical molecules by polyinosinic acid and polyadenylic acid. *Nature*, 181(4608), 521–525.

Ristanis, S., Giakas, G., Papageorgiou, C.D., Moraiti, T., Stergiou, N., Georgoulis, A.D. (2003). The effects of anterior cruciate ligament reconstruction on tibial rotation during pivoting after descending stairs. *Knee Surgery Sports Traumatology and Arthroscopy*, 11(6), 360–365.

Ristanis, S., Stergiou, N., Patras, K., Tsepis, E., Moraiti, C., Georgoulis, A.D. (2006). Follow-up evaluation 2 years after ACL reconstruction with bone-patellar tendon-bone graft shows that excessive tibial rotation persists. *Clinical Journal of Sports Medicine*, 16(2), 111–116.

Ristanis, S., Stergiou, N., Patras, K., Vasiliadis, H.S., Giakas, G., Georgoulis, A.D. (2005). Excessive tibial rotation during high-demand activities is not restored by anterior cruciate ligament reconstruction. *Arthroscopy*, 21(11), 1323–1329.

Ristanis, S., Stergiou, N., Siarava, E., Ntoulia, A., Mitsionis, G., Georgoulis, A. D. (2009). Effect of femoral tunnel placement for reconstruction of the anterior cruciate ligament on tibial rotation. *The Journal of Bone and Joint Surgery*, 91(9), 2151–2158.

Sherrington, C.S. (1898). Decerebrate rigidity and reflex coordination of movements. *Journal of Physiology*, 22, 319–332.

Sherrington, C.S. (1906). *Integrative Action of the Nervous System*. New York: Scribner.

Shik, M.L., Severin, F.V., Orlovsky, G.N. (1966). Control of walking and running by means of electrical stimulation of the mid-brain. *Biophysics*, 11, 756–765.

Smith, B.L., Thelen, E. (1994). *A Dynamic Systems Approach to Development. Applications*. Cambridge, MA: MIT Press.

Stergiou, N., Ristanis, S., Moraiti, C., Georgoulis, A.D. (2007). Tibial rotation in anterior cruciate ligament (ACL)-deficient and ACL-reconstructed knees: a theoretical proposition for the development of osteoarthritis. *Sports Medicine*, 37(7), 601–613.

Taub, E., Berman, A.J. (1968). Movement and learning in the absence of sensory feedback. In S.J. Freedman (Ed.), *The Neurophysiology of Spatially Oriented Behavior* (pp. 173–192). Homewood, NJ: Dorsey Press.

Thelen, E. (1986). Treadmill-elicited stepping in seven-month-old infants. *Child Development*, 57, 1498–1506.

Thelen, E., Fisher, D.M., Ridley-Johnson, R. (1984). The relationship between physical growth and a newborn reflex. *Infant Behavior and Development*, 7, 479–493.

Thelen, E., Ulrich, B.D. (1991). Hidden skills: a dynamic analysis of treadmill stepping during the first year. *Monographs of the Society for Research in Child Development*, 56(1), 1–98.Thelen, E., Ulrich, B.D., Niles, D. (1987). Bilateral coordination in human infants: stepping on a split-belt treadmill. *Journal of Experimental Psychology: Human Perception and Performance*, 13, 405–410.

Watson, J.D., Crick, F.H. (1953). Molecular structure of nucleic acids: a structure for deoxyribose nucleic acid. *Nature*, 171(4356), 73–78.

Woollacott, M.H., Jensen, J. (1996). Posture and locomotion. In H. Heuer & S. Keele (Eds.), *Handbook of Perception and Action* (2nd Edition, pp. 303–403). New York: Academic Press.

chapter two

Getting your grant proposals funded

> Science is built up with facts, as a house is with stones. But a collection of facts is no more a science than a heap of stones is a house.

—Jules Henri Poincaré (1854–1912)

2.1   Introduction

This chapter provides a comprehensive approach with numerous examples and tips on how to get your grant proposals funded. In addition, it provides tips on organizing and producing a successful research plan with novel ideas; the foundation for good grantsmanship.

2.2   Why is grant writing important?

Regardless of whether you go in to industry or academia, and regardless of what you may do eventually, you will almost always need to be able to get financial support for your endeavors. For this purpose, you will have to carefully craft successful proposals. This is even more important today because the available funds, especially for research in academia, have decreased in recent years. This has happened for two reasons. There is a larger demand for research funds by the increased number of scientists competing for them. In addition, the available research funds have not kept up with the demand. For example, on average, only 10% of applications get funded, at least at the National Institutes of Health (NIH), when a few decades ago, this number was 30% or higher. Thus, there is a limited amount of funding available, and it is very competitive. I received my first NIH grant only after I tried multiple attempts, and if we measure my success rate early in my career in terms of applying for grants, it is truly pitiful. Success requires a tremendous amount of patience and persistence. So, a natural questions arises: If the odds are so low, why should I spend my time writing grants? Let me give you some very good reasons.

1. *You can get research personnel.* Imagine how difficult it would be as a young human movement scientist in academia to find subjects, bring them to the laboratory, set up the laboratory, collect all the data, process it, run the statistics, and write the paper. Imagine how long it will take if you have to do everything by yourself. This in addition to all other responsibilities you may have (i.e. teaching, service). A single paper requires a year or more of hard work. This is exactly what I was doing for the first 4–5 years of my career, and my research productivity was very low. You need funding to be able to hire research personnel in order to be more efficient and explore all the wonderful hypotheses you have in your laboratory notebook.

2. *You can conduct larger research projects.* For example, in human movement research that is clinically oriented, you will almost never be able to perform a clinical trial if you do not have funds. Your research will be limited in its reach and scope.

3. *You can stay employed.* In academic fields, and in many other institutions, you need to get funding to get continuation and to receive tenure. In my situation, one of the things that happened when I received my first large federal grant is that I was able to get a much bigger laboratory. My first laboratory space was a small room, and my main piece of instrumentation, a force platform, was installed on the floor in a space next to mine. I had to book that space for data collection, which also meant I had to move the rest of my equipment in and out of the room each time I used it. Unfortunately, this space was used as a classroom, and that meant moving all of the teaching equipment as well. However, the worst part was that it was available only during late Fridays and weekends. So, when I received the federal grant, I went to my Chair and said, "so what would you like me to do? I have got to collect all of these data to do the work I proposed." He replied, "I don't know." So, I said, "maybe I should decline all this money." He immediately rejected this proposition and dedicated that space to my research. Now why did he do that? What does the university get out of it?
   - First, more prestige...
   - Second, more students (another measure of success is the number of credit-hours students enroll in), and...
   - Third, more *money* (see Vignette 2.1).

That is why institutions require you to receive funding in order to get tenure.

VIGNETTE 2.1   Direct and indirect costs

Indirect cost is extremely important for every institution. Grant funding includes both direct and indirect costs. *Direct cost* is the money that is received to actually perform the research. For example, in order to perform a certain experiment, I need graduate students and a piece of instrumentation, both of which I write into my budget. If my budget turns out to be $1 million, the university charges another half a million dollars on the top of that. Why? Because there are other necessary things that are needed in order for you to be able to perform the experiment. For example, you need lights and heat to be able to work, the room needs to be clean, and so on. This does not only apply to the laboratory; it applies to the library and many other resources that the university provides for you to do your work; like administration, personnel, and security costs. This is why the university needs to charge the extra money that is called the indirect cost. At my institution, indirect cost is currently 46.5% of the direct cost. At other institutions, it could be more. For example, at the University of Colorado it is 54%, and at Massachusetts Institute of Technology (MIT) it is 54.7% (www.colorado.edu/controller/about/general-accounting/cost-accounting; http://web.mit.edu/fnl/volume/295/zuber.html). Now in some universities, some of the indirect cost comes back to the department and to the faculty members. For example, when I established our Department of Biomechanics, I successfully negotiated for us to receive almost 50% of the indirect cost that we generate. This is how we finance graduate and undergraduate students and support many other functions of our department.

---

4. *You are considered successful.* It is not too difficult to publish scientific articles. You only need to convince a few reviewers in order for your research to be accepted. But how difficult is to get funding to support your research, especially when we are talking about millions of dollars? In order to receive funding, you have to convince a large number of reviewers, a whole study section, which often comprises the best scientists in the field. Once you have money, you can hire more research personnel and conduct more research, which becomes an important measure of success. Back to the money draw, you also become very marketable once you are successfully funded. Institutions value people who bring them money and may even head hunt them.

And my last, but most important reason for writing grants…

5. *Your research ideas are peer-reviewed.* Writing a grant has a major benefit to *you*. It allows you to organize your thoughts in terms of strong inference (see chapter one). It forces you to put your thoughts together on paper and organize them as a logical tree of sequential experiments. It gives you the drive to create crucial experiments and test hypotheses that will disprove your theory. You advance your reasoning, and you get your ideas into a more concrete, thorough, and comprehensive document. Then, "it allows you to have your thoughts and ideas tested". Established scientists will read your ideas and review them. You will receive feedback that states whether your ideas are worth pursuing. Often, you will receive a critique that you can use to improve your strong inference.

As a young scientist, you might think that you have great ideas. However, do other scientists share your enthusiasm? Are your ideas worth funding? Imagine someone comes to you and asks for your opinion of their work. You'll help them if you have the time. Now imagine if they ask you for money so that they may pursue their work. The stakes become higher because money is involved. You will have to look very critically at their ideas. This is exactly why agencies appoint established scientists to evaluate your ideas. You will receive honest feedback from these professionals because money is involved; either your ideas are worthy or unworthy of their funding. When I started my career, I applied for funds to do research on my ideas with respect to running injuries. Running mechanics was a big part of my PhD, and I thought that running injuries were very important. Another perspective never occurred to me. However, when people are injured, they can stop running and do other sports; swimming or biking, etc. That is fundamental. There are other problems like multiple sclerosis and stroke; problems that affect basic mobility. You can't ask patients with those more serious problems to "start doing other sports." Who provided me with the lecture that prompted that change in heart? A Program Officer from the NIH. He asked me why I was wasting my life and told me to get serious and put my talent to good use. "Do something that will actually touch peoples' lives," he said. With my running ideas, I wasn't going anywhere as the funding institutions simply did not find them worthy of their funds as there are much more important problems in society that need financial support. From that point on, I started working in clinical biomechanics, and I translated my theoretical perspective to ask questions that could touch people's lives.

2.3   Motivation for grant writing

When writing grants, there are really two main types of motivation:

Extrinsic motivation: Motivation from incentives (money, awards, perks). Here are a few examples. As faculty, you are most often employed on a 9-month contract. What will you do in the summer? Go paint houses as some of my colleagues were doing when I started at my institution? Absolutely not! You have so much talent, you worked so hard to gain invaluable knowledge, and, of course, you will put it to good use. So, why wouldn't you write some grants and buy that time? In addition, many institutions have what is called overload. If you can buy all your time and your summer, you can go above the money you make into your contract. At some institutions, you can go up to 50%. In addition, your grant funding could allow you to travel.[1] You also get prestige. Slowly, you establish yourself, you do bigger projects, you get more people, and you publish more papers. People will start to invite you to speak or collaborate and want to know how you became successful. And, of course, they pay for your travel expenses.

Intrinsic motivation: Motivation from the enjoyment of doing the task or for the feeling of accomplishment. Several studies have indicated that faculty members are more driven by intrinsic rather than extrinsic motivation (Hardre et al., 2011; Smith, 2016). It is the feeling of self-worth, satisfaction, happiness, confidence, and the feeling of success. This is definitely my personal motivation.

2.4   Where is the money?

There are many funding agencies to apply for research funding. At the *Federal level*, for example, there are the NIH, the National Science Foundation (NSF), and many other institutions. I personally believe that the reason that the United States is so successful in terms of research and innovation is because of the NSF and NIH. In fact, a lot of funding institutions around the world have tried to imitate their model. Researchers compete for a large amount of money, allowing the most promising and innovative ideas to be pursued. One of the major accomplishments of the NIH is the increase of the life expectancy in the United States by at least 10 years. In addition, every governmental department has a research entity or institute within it. For example, the Department of Defense has its own research department. The Veterans' Administration also has their own research department. You can certainly apply to them and receive funding to pursue your ideas.

There is also state-based funding for research. A very good example in my state is the Nebraska Research Initiative. Some of the state tax dollars goes into this entity. This budget is handled by the President of the

---

[1] When I came to my institution I was given only $500 in travel funds. I remember I went to the American Society of Biomechanics meeting in my very first year. I shared a room with another young scientist who I didn't know beforehand. Unfortunately, he snored loudly! I don't believe I slept for several days. This is all that I could do with that amount of money; share a room. I couldn't travel internationally, of course.

University of Nebraska, who has initiated many wonderful programs. For example, in 2016 there was a program named *Food for Health*. One of my first large grants that I received was a state grant. Here you are only competing against people from the same state and the odds could be better. In addition, certain states are eligible for IDeA (Institutional Development Award) funding from the NIH or are considered EPSCoR (Experimental Program to Stimulate Competitive Research) from the NSF, NASA, and others (www.nigms.nih.gov/Research/DRCB/IDeA/Pages/default.aspx; www.nsf.gov/od/oia/programs/epscor/). The IDeA program enhances research capacities in states that historically have had low levels of NIH funding by supporting basic, clinical, and translational research; faculty development; and infrastructure improvements. EPSCoR enhances research competitiveness of targeted jurisdictions (states, territories, and commonwealth) by strengthening STEM (science, technology, engineering, and mathematics) capacity and capability.

Then there are private agencies. What do I mean by *private* funds? Well, wealthy people create foundations to provide money for research. The Gates foundation, the Michael J. Fox foundation, and others provide private funds. All of my research on multiple sclerosis was funded by the MARS foundation. There are many others out there.

Regarding all these funding sources, I want to give you some advice. *Diversify your portfolio.* By that, I mean the NIH is not the only funding agency out there. *Go after everyone that will listen to you.* I know people who made their career receiving funding from the NIH. However, what happens if something goes wrong with this specific source? If you don't get continuation of your grants (at least in big universities), you've lost all your funding, and you have to fire everybody from your laboratory. You will lose your trusted technicians, graduate students won't come to you because you cannot support them, and you're back to trying to do all your experiments by yourself. In addition, get your graduate students to buy into the mentality that everybody needs to help with funding. They can also apply for fellowships, travel grants, and others to support their laboratory. Writing grants to receive funding from different sources will not only help you improve your rationale and your logic but also improve your CV.

2.5 Tips for successful proposals for any funding agency

The first and most important tip to write successful proposals is to be organized. For this purpose, I personally use what I call the seven-step approach. I want to give credit for this approach to Dr. Carol Nicholson at the NIH and the National Institute of Child Health and Human Development (NICHD) who gave me an initial layout of the seven steps.

2.5.1   Step 1: Create your grant's notebook

You can either have a hard copy notebook or an electronic one. If it's hard copy, get a *BIG one* with dividers where you include the following:

Application form and guidelines. Hint: Before you apply, do a thorough search for any guidelines that you can find.

The agency's mission. Hint: You have to make sure that your purpose fits their needs. It's not the other way around.

Contact information and anything you can find out about the reviewers. Hint: Compile everything that you can find out about the people that will judge your grant. For example, we know the reviewers at the NIH. If they are in your area of study, make sure that you don't omit important references that are co-authors. Try to get them to know you as well. Go to meetings that they attend and introduce yourself; of course never mention your proposal, as they will not be able to discuss it with you. Read the articles they have published and visit their websites to get to know them (Vignette 2.2.).

Previously funded applications of the agency. Hint: Often, you can find what these agencies have funded in the past. This will tell you if your research will be something that will be interested in supporting.

Timeline to check your progress. You need a very long timeline to fit in everything you need to do. If anyone thinks that you can decide to apply for a grant and get everything done in 10 days, then they are deluded. You have to set a timeline.

VIGNETTE 2.2   Satisfying the reviewers – a side story

I had submitted a grant to the NIH and received a decent score, but it was not funded. Based on the comments, I thought that there might be a chance it would get funded if I resubmitted it. One of the comments asked me to add a consultant in a specific area of study, but I wasn't sure which person would be best for this consultancy. I went through the roster of the reviewers. I knew one of the reviewers listed on there by reputation and suspected that this person was one of my reviewers. I went to the reviewer's website and discovered that the reviewer will be attending that year a specific meeting. I targeted that meeting and submitted a poster. Having found out what the reviewer looked like from the internet, I found the reviewer at the meeting, introduced myself and complimented the work that was performed in the reviewer's laboratory. The reviewer thanked me and asked me about my work. I presented my work and handed copies of my poster.[2] I then asked the question I had come for but in a completely indirect way. I said that I have a professional question, and I would like some advice. On a grant that I wrote, a reviewer had asked me to add a consultant that had expertise in this area. I asked, "Do you know of who such a person might be?" The reviewer recommended a specific individual. I called this person, and I was able to add this expert as a consultant on the grant. The grant was funded on the next round, and I feel this helped. Every little thing helps, and such little things can put your grant over the top.

2.5.2   Step 2: Getting you and your science ready for review

Write one page with your hypotheses/aims and the significance of your study with respect to the mission of the agency. Hint: Don't forget strong inference. You don't need to write a lot; only one page. Maybe write four paragraphs that explain why this is an important problem, how your ideas are linked with the problem and your hypothesis, and then the significance of your study with the respect to the mission of the agency.

Email this page to the agency to receive feedback. Hint: Some agencies require something like that to pre-screen you. They call it a *letter of intent*. Some agencies do not provide feedback. Do not be disappointed if you don't get any feedback, as long as your ideas fit well with the mission of the agency.

Email this page to a few trusted colleagues that can give honest feedback. Hint: Trusted colleagues means those who will be willing to tell you the truth and will not steal your ideas.

Tighten your aims based on the feedback you receive. Hint: Read this feedback carefully, and if you need to restart with a new "logical tree," do so. Remember that your ego is in your garbage can.

2.5.3   Step 3: Look at the scientific mandates of the work you propose

The science has to be startling, clear, and compelling.

If you are not a biostatistician yourself, obtain formal professional biostatistical help, giving the biostatistician the research aims. Hint: You should have a

---

[2] Don't go to a meeting without a print out of your poster because you do more presenting in the hallways than you do standing in front of it.

very good relationship with a biostatistician. That doesn't mean that you don't have to take statistics in graduate school. How many statistics course I have taken? I took eight! Who has been teaching advanced statistics in our department for years? I have. I still use a biostatistician. Why? Because a biostatistician does this job every day, I don't. Ask for a power analysis and a synopsis of the biostatistical modeling/analysis that will be used. Make sure you understand the concepts well, so that it is easier to formulate a research plan.

Read and reread the world's literature, paying special attention to studies similar to yours. Hint: You need to be extremely knowledgeable of the literature in your field; you need to have depth and breadth in terms of your knowledge (chapter one). Include literature that goes back 100 years, or more, if needed. You may need to read things from other disciplines as well, if they are related to what you are doing.[3]

2.5.4 Step 4: Making a grant proposal

Make a very detailed outline of your research plan. Hint: Questions, such as how you will collect subjects, who will be the collaborating clinician, who will help recruit the subjects, and what are the inclusion and exclusion criteria, are extremely important. Based on your subject population, you need to examine if your proposed work is feasible before you start. I once had a graduate student who wanted to do his dissertation on a very specific patient population. He had no idea of the feasibility of what he was proposing. He had no clinical collaborators. I had my reservations, but I reluctantly agreed. He ended up gathering only five subjects over a 2-year period, and the study was a massive failure. On the other hand, a more recent student of mine who was, however, a clinician, was able to gather 30 subjects from the same patient population in the same period of time. Because of my experience with the first one, I was extremely skeptical, but the student demonstrated feasibility and eventually the study came through.

Give the aims, the power analysis, and the detailed outline to a senior, funded researcher at your institution who is not politically connected to you in any way. Hint: Ask for a harsh criticism and ask for any suggestions. Give the senior researcher a full 3 weeks to do it. You should give your aims to someone

---

[3] Even if you think you know the entire literature extremely well, never write in your publication "this is the first paper...." If you write "this is the first paper," there is always a chance a knowledgeable reviewer will send you the paper that was truly the first paper and you will be so embarrassed!

who is not politically connected to you. It is highly important to ask for harsh criticism in order to attain genuine feedback.[4]

Get the Institutional Review Board (IRB) application together, and line up letters of support. Hint: You need a letter of support from your department chair who is in charge of the laboratories and of your time. For example, if the grant requires you devote 75% of your time to research and your chair can only afford to give you 50%, you will have a major problem. As another example, if you are going to be using an MRI machine or patients from a different institution, you need to provide a letter of support from that department that proves you have the access to that environment. If you are using a biostatistician, you need a letter of support. You also need to finish the IRB application.

Start writing the entire grant, following the directions in your notebook very carefully. Hint: As you begin to write, keep in mind the purpose of the program announcement of the specific agency and whatever evaluation criteria are available. You also need to follow the writing directions of the specific agency you're applying for. Every agency has their own writing directions. The NIH, for example, has directions regarding the space between sentences on the page, fonts, and other very specific requirements. You need to follow their directions to the letter. You must read and reread the agency mission because you have to remember that "you are not writing the grant for yourself, but for the agency". The grant has to fit the mission and the evaluation criteria of the agency.

2.5.5   Step 5: An application emerges…

When the critiqued outline is back from the senior researcher (don't forget a thank you note), make a grant out of it.

Complete a draft of the entire proposal, including the budget. Hint: You should allow eight full weeks for this transition.

Now you have a draft. Hint: You can ask the scientist who helped you to take another look and your colleagues, too. At the end of this time, your proposal should look like a grant. Follow the instructions in your notebook carefully and adhere to page limits.

---

[4] I remember this wonderful man who read the very first grant that I wrote. I was very proud of writing my first grant. However, I wanted to get feedback. Then, I didn't know many people at my institution and hardly anyone was writing NIH grants. So, I went to the Sponsored Projects Office, and I presented my very first grant, my *masterpiece*, to Dr. Glenn Dalrymple who was a radiologist from our Medical School and he used to sit on study sections at the NIH. He asked me to sit down and told me, "you don't have any idea about writing grants." He then threw my masterpiece in the garbage! I actually had tears in my eyes as I considered how hard I had worked and how unprepared I was. However, I was determined and tenacious. So, I humbly asked him to guide me on how to write grants. He smiled and said to me, "ok let's do it." Then he started teaching me how to write grants, line by line…

Do not over budget or under budget in your proposal. Hint: Reviewers will question your justification and your grant could be rejected. If you under budget, you could look naïve. For example, I do not have a lot of time to spend on research projects. If I state that I will dedicate 5% of my time to my grant, they'll wonder if I'm serious about my work. If you over budget, you may look greedy. When you are formulating your budget, you need to think carefully about what you need (supplies, personnel, publication fees, etc.), and how you can fit your needs within the guidelines of the specific agency to which you are applying. Grant mechanisms usually have maximum amounts of funds for which you can apply.

Get people to read your whole grant. Hint: I have one of my staff members who has a BSc in General Studies to read my grants. She should be able to understand it, otherwise I am writing in a very complex way that reviewers may not be able to understand either. Simplicity in writing is a great virtue. Also, since I am international, I always ask someone to check my English. You have to listen to your readers and make their suggested changes.

Now you have a grant! Hint: Review the instructions, check the formatting, check the page limits, and

PUT IT AWAY...

After at least a 5-day break, look at the grant again, and tune and tweak. Hint: Get your institutional and departmental signoffs. Chip away at your IRB submission, so that it is ready to turn in the week before your review (or sooner). You do NOT have to have IRB approval before you send in the grant, but they will not release the funds to you until you have this.

2.5.6 Step 6: Get that grant out!

Compose the cover letter. Hint: It is extremely important to submit a good cover letter.[5] You can write and explain the specifics of your grant. Why did you want to submit to this agency? What have you done in terms of the procedures? Include sentences from the mission as well. If possible, get feedback from the agency on this letter.

Ten days before the due date, submit it!!...

Five days later, make sure it is at the funding agency office. Hint: Put it in a drawer for a while but keep attending to the literature. Make 100% sure that your ideas have not already been done.

After review, you will receive a Summary Statement (see more on this later). Hint: Go over your comments with program staff, who will also be able

---

[5] I write cover letters for everything. For example, when I submit a manuscript, I add a cover letter with it (more on this will be discussed later). I know a lot of people who send their papers out to journals without a cover letter, then they wonder why their papers are rejected.

to give you guidance regarding the likelihood of funding at this point, or after resubmission. It is very important to get sound feedback on this. If the comments are *constructive*, then you have a higher likelihood of being approved by the agency. If the comments are *lukewarm* ("The rationale is unclear," "there is potential, but we are not certain how things will be done," "I'm not 100% sure of the big picture") then I recommend starting to look for other agencies or to start over, possibly from scratch. Make sure that you do not get angry when you receive comments from the grant reviewers if your proposal is rejected. I know people who have started yelling at the Program Officer because their grants were either rejected or received bad reviews. This is a terrible mistake. Take a time out, then go back to the comments and see if you can address them calmly.

2.5.7   Step 7: REST, don't quit, REST, don't quit!

Do not quit, it will happen. You just have to be persistent. Hint: You will fail many times at first and you should know that if you are successful on your first try, then you will fail on your next ten.

"*Success is not final, and failure is not fatal: it is the courage to continue that counts." – Winston Churchill.* Hint: Just like I told you before, my first ten or so federal grant applications were rejected. You will have many disappointments before you make it. If you have to do rewrites, wait until you have digested the comments in the Summary Statement. Read them yourself. Ask a senior researcher to review them with you. It is very important to get other peoples' perspectives.

2.6   Tips for getting funding

Below I have compiled several more tips for getting your grants funded.

Make sure you have the support of your chairman. You will need resources from the university to do your research. They will be given to you if you work hard and you are a team player. I always helped my chairman in anything he asked of me, and I knew that he appreciated my willingness to help at crucial times that he needed help.

Make sure you know what your development office can do for you and gain their support (use chocolate). The development office are usually the people who submit the grants. In my institution, they also help me to develop my budget. Every year, around Christmas time, I buy a lot of chocolate, and I hand it to the development office staff. I have been doing this for 15–20 years. They always remember the chocolate, and I feel that this gesture has always helped me with how my grants are treated in their office.

Build your facilities and equipment using foundation and other internal grants. I recommend against asking for basic equipment through federal grants. It will look like you don't have the resources to perform your experiments. However, to have a strong and supportive environment is always part of the evaluation criteria. This is why you need to obtain your equipment and build your facilities using internal mechanisms such as funds from the university's foundation. When such opportunities arise, make sure you go after them with fervor. A solid presentation of your needs could be very effective.[6]

Develop a focused line of research using strong inference. Try not to do everything at the same time. You should have one line of research or a well-developed logical tree. However, you should also make sure that you have a couple of different lines of research or couple of other logical trees you have developed at least in a conceptual basis, in case you reach a dead end with the one you are pursuing at the moment. Two or three lines of research is a decent number but not several. That will exhaust your energy.

Graduate student research projects should fall within the focus of your research. Graduate students should pursue experimental work that is similar to yours and contribute to your logical tree. Eventually, they can branch out on they own but initially need to work closely to you. In this fashion, the eventual publications will provide you important preliminary data and will allow you to strengthen your CV, demonstrating credibility. If the graduate students want to perform work that is outside your area of study, you will not be able to help them intimately, and, again, you will be losing too much energy trying to supervise them. Remember they came to work with you and not the other way around.

Every study should have a high potential for publication (be a finisher). Are you sending your publications only to *Science* and *Nature*? I hope not. Some of your publications will be in very good journals, some of them will be in journals of lesser impact. However, the most important thing is to get your work out there in order to be read. My PhD mentor has always said that his best publication was one that he wrote with me that

---

[6] When I started my career, I did not have high-speed cameras (an essential piece of equipment to do my research), and we only had cameras that ran at 30 frames per second. I actually had to rent cameras. The rent was $500 per day which was very expensive for me at that time. So, I would rent them and collect data over the weekend like a madman. The weekend gave me two extra days with the cameras. Finally, I had an opportunity to purchase high-speed cameras from a specific internal mechanism. I went to present my case in front of a panel of university officials. The total amount I was asking was $50K. In my presentation, I handed them a little mouse that you wind up and it performs a front flip. I then played two videos I'd recorded, one of which was captured with our old 30 Hz camera, and the other with a high-speed camera. In the 30 Hz recording, my mouse was a disjointed blur. With the high-speed camera, you could see the entire flip in vivid detail. I then asked them which one was a better device to use to analyze the movement. They all answered, "the second." I replied, "Right now, we have the first and all I am asking you is to provide me with the money to buy the second." I got the funds!

was published in an obscure journal called *Journal of Human Movement Studies* (Bates and Stergiou, 1996). It took us forever to publish that paper because a lot of people did not believe the results. They made perfect sense, but people did not believe them. However, eventually our ideas broke through and were accepted by others. The seminal publication of Edward Lorenz in 1963 that practically introduced Chaos theory, did not immediately attract attention beyond Lorenz' own field. It was published in the *Journal of the Atmospheric Sciences* that was of lesser impact and not widely read. But, by the mid-1970s, with the rise of similar work by Benoit Mandelbrot and others, the term "butterfly effect" that was introduced by Lorenz, had become a subject of debate which seemed to affect a wide range of academic disciplines, and the Lorenz's paper began to be cited regularly (Lorenz, 1963).

Develop relationships and collaborations (clinicians, biostatisticians, engineers, etc.). You have to *talk to people* and market your research. Be social and leave your comfort zone. Go to conferences. Present your work. Introduce yourself and engage with other scientists. Every time I went to the American Society of Biomechanics meeting, I used to contact a senior person in my field ahead of time to have breakfast or lunch together. The purpose was to learn from their wisdom. In one of my such meetings as a faculty member, I sent an email to Dr. Walter Herzog and asked him to breakfast. He provided me with excellent ideas on how to run my laboratory, which I am still using today. Attend the business meetings at conferences. It will put you right in the heart of the society.[7] Nowadays, I also use social media to attract more people to my work.

Attend university events, parties, and seminars. Ask people to lunch or coffee. Try to take advantage of every opportunity that is available to you. My good friend and collaborator, Dr. Dmitry Oleynikov, and I worked together for many years on minimally invasive surgery using my ideas on variability from a learning perspective. I was helping him to develop ways to teach surgeons how to use surgical robots. We have published almost 20 papers together. That helped me improve my CV as a young scientist, doing meaningful impactful research. We were also able to receive significant amount of funding that supported our laboratories. Our first grant was for $2 million. Well, I met Dr. Oleynikov at a party!

The scientific quality of a project determines whether it is funded. If you don't have a really good idea (solid hypotheses with crucial experiments), your project will not get funded. Everything else is the icing on the cake

---

[7] I am one of the editors in the *Journal of Biomechanics*. How did I get this position? I attended one of the business meetings of the American Society of Biomechanics. The President asked for a few people to sit on the editorial board and represent the society, and I volunteered. By doing this sort of thing, you improve your reputation and more people will know of you.

(getting the consultants, working the politics of the science, etc.). This is why strong inference is so important.

The presentation of your application can make or break your application (typos, grammar, inconsistencies, etc.). Be very careful with your writing presentation when you are submitting any type of application (even emails).[8] Be meticulous. In general, if you're not meticulous you cannot be a scientist. There is no room for sloppiness in science.

For all agencies, good grantsmanship is knowing how to identify the "hot buttons" that need to be punched, and then knowing how to punch them! In order to identify the hot buttons, you need to examine what each specific agency wants in the future. You need to evaluate carefully not only its mission statement, but also their annual report and especially their strategic planning. You might also go to meetings and talk to the agencies. A great meeting to do so is the annual conference of the Society for Neuroscience where many agencies have booths and there are plenty of program officers available to answer questions.

2.7 Assess your grant application

Reviewers will assess whether you have the resources to get the job done (bricks). They will assess everything: the entire environment, the facilities, the equipment, your letters of support, etc. They will assess if you have the required equipment to do the study. I spoke about this above but here I want to stress that, when you apply for a position at a new university, you should ask for start-up funds to acquire the instrumentation needed.[9] They will also assess if your institution allows sufficient time to perform your research. Your chair must provide assurances that you will have sufficient release to dedicate time to research.

Reviewers will assess whether you and your institution have the expertise to get the job done (brains). Reviewers will assess if you are a *credible individual*. First, they will assess you through the papers that you have published. A good number of publications in peer-reviewed journals will suggest that you are both a hard worker and a finisher. Second, they will examine your CV for pertinent work. You should be able to show evidence that you have worked and delivered in the same field as the grant for which

---

[8] On a related note, be very careful when sending an email to a professor you want to be your mentor for your PhD or postdoc. Do you think you will be accepted if you make orthographical mistakes during that *first impression* email? You didn't even have time to check your spelling mistakes? That is sloppiness. No one will want to work with you if your work is riddled with errors.

[9] This is also important for graduate students applying for PhD positions and for PhD students applying for a postdoc. Is the equipment that you need to perform my experiments available? If you apply to a university that doesn't have the required equipment to allow you to do your job, you will be in trouble.

you are applying. Are you, the Principal Investigator, and your colleagues qualified to do the work? If a doctoral student of yours is submitting an F31 (doctoral fellowship) application, they will not know the candidate. However, they will assess you as the mentor. Are you qualified? Have you demonstrated that you can publish and be productive? You are required to establish yourself and become known by "paving your way with publications". It is critical to publish in order to establish your credibility. As we said above, aim to publish high-quality research articles but do not concentrate on high impact journals all the time. Maybe smaller projects will lead to bigger ones in the future. Sometimes you will not even know the impact that a publication will have. One of the top five papers I published (in terms of citations) was extremely simple but part of solid reasoning (chapter one; examples of strong inference). We collected data from anterior cruciate ligament-injured individuals who also had a reconstruction. We collected the data in Greece, with low cost equipment and using only kinematic variables. Several years later I was listening to Dr. Thomas P. Andriacchi, one of the most prominent biomechanists in the field of sport medicine and orthopedics, delivering his acceptance speech of the Borelli award at the American Society of Biomechanics. This is the most prestigious award of the Society. I was massively surprised when he praised our paper as the crucial paper that led him to his new line of research and the theoretical perspective he was using at that time. Thus, the point here is that sometimes you might think that a study is not important, but it could have a major impact on the field. Don't let data sit around collecting dust.

Assess yourself.[10] Before you move forward with this novel idea, assess yourself.

- Do you have the expertise?
- Do you have the resources?
- Do you have the personnel?
- Do you have the preliminary data to be competitive?

Assess the competition. Before you move forward with your idea, assess the competition through the literature and databases of existing grants. Looking through grant databases is very important. Is your project or something very similar being done currently?[11] For example, the NIH has

---

[10] The Program Officer who told me to stop researching running injuries made me realize that it might be more profitable (and valuable) for me to look into osteoarthritis, which could be the outcome of running injuries. He then asked me why he should fund me instead of Thomas P. Andriacchi. He meant that there are a lot of other really good people that I need to compete with.

[11] Looking at the databases can also give you an indication of the types of research each agency has funded in the past – does yours fit in?

an excellent database called the RePORTER (https://projectreporter.nih. gov/reporter.cfm). The NSF also has a powerful database www.nsf.gov/ awardsearch/).

Assess the agency. Grants exist for the sole purpose of having the applicant help the funding agency achieve its mission. *You propose research to help the agency fulfill its mission and not the other way around!* The NIH reports directly to the government. Funding agencies such as the Christopher Reeve Foundation have a board of directors. Every year the program officers need to prepare an annual report and deliver it to the board. Their report needs to clearly outline that they have spent their funds to the best interest of the agency. Therefore, find the agency that has a mission that fits your idea; that is, where your research will help the agency to achieve its goals. Both the idea and the funding agency must be considered hand-in-hand. Your idea will not be a good fit for all agencies. For example, the NIH has several institutes and each one has its own focus. If you have an idea related to bioengineering, the National Institute of Biomedical Imaging and Bioengineering (NIBIB) may be interested. If your project deals with stroke, the National Institute of Neurological Disorders and Stroke (NINDS) may be a good fit. Contact the Program Officer about your idea and listen carefully to the advice you are given.

Assess your idea. Your idea is key, and everything hinges on strong inference. Sometimes graduate students have several ideas and cannot contain them. Others have a problem with creating ideas. The answer is always in the methodical application of strong inference. For graduate students, first you have to identify the specific area of research that you will focus on. At the beginning you might have just an inclination, a desire to solve a specific problem that possibly affects you. Maybe your grandmother fell down, which lead to a major health deficit, and you decided to help her. This is why you want to start working on loss of balance in older adults. You can develop multiple ideas but do not force it. Read massively and add the results to your logical tree. Most of the time, the idea comes out of nowhere.

Young (2003) suggested the following five steps to developing a novel idea.

- Gather its raw material – read the literature massively.
- Masticate and organize this material.
- Put the subject away for a while.
- Out of nowhere the idea will appear – the *Eureka!* moment.[12]
- Check how the idea fares in the world and refine it.

---

[12] Usually the best ideas, the crucial experiments for me, do not come overnight. I organize everything I read in my laboratory notebook and then put it aside. Eventually one day I wake up, when walking to my car or when I am at the shower, and the idea pops up. The Eureka moment will only happen this way.

Russell and Morrison (2016) expanded the above steps in six steps.

- Define the problem or need that you want to address (do not forget strong inference).
- Collect and critically analyze the literature.
- Generate a preliminary idea.
- Assess the idea's potential for success and modify it if necessary.
  - Will this idea impact significantly on my field?
  - If so, can I convince others of this fact?
  - Can I do it? Do I have the ability? Do I have the resources?
  - Critically assess the competition.
- Seek constructive criticism of your idea from knowledgeable colleagues.
- Refine the idea to maximize its potential for impact in your field.

It would be rare for an individual with a good idea to be unable to identify at least one funding agency interested in supporting it. If you have a good idea, you will be funded one way or another. You need to be persistent. After you come up with an idea, you should seek feedback. A more experienced individual may give you guidance on whether the idea has potential. You need to be careful of who you present your ideas to. You need to trust this individual. How do we trust someone? Trust comes from the positive recommendations and references that you receive from friends and colleagues. When you receive feedback and criticism, you should incorporate it and refine the idea based on the comments you receive.

2.8   Research advance: At Pitt, scientists decode the secret of getting grants – marketing helps university win $350 million a year from the NIH

This article, which was published in *The Wall Street Journal* in 2004, has several interesting messages regarding how to be successful in acquiring grants (Wysocki, 2004). The article presents the approach of Dr. David Kupfer, then Head of Psychiatry at the University of Pittsburg. I would like to highlight here some aspects of his approach.

- Being in a Department of Psychiatry, his target agency was the NIH. Dr. Kupfer spoke continuously with NIH officials about hot new areas that might produce funding for his faculty and other scientists.
- He required that all young scientists attend "boot camps" on grant writing.

- It was important to him that his scientists get to sit on NIH study sections to better understand the grant reviewing mechanisms.
- He incentivized success in grant funding by giving "bonuses" of as much as $50,000 each time they received a NIH grant.
- He ran an intensive "survival skills" course for young postdoctoral fellows in psychiatry to train them in the fine points of applying for their first grants.
- He asked his young scientists to learn to focus their proposals more narrowly.
- He also taught his young scientists the value of marketing or branding. He wanted them to think about what they would write on their "research t-shirt" or a quick catchy phrase that tells the world what their research stands for.

As a Chair in my department, I have adopted, at different levels, all of the above. I require that my young faculty members and postdocs attend grant writing workshops, and I recommend they sit on study sections of different agencies. With the help of my university's foundation, I have also implemented a "bonus" mechanism when they get a federal grant. I run a 7 AM every-Thursday seminar on how to write grants every Fall that all doctoral students, postdocs, and young faculty are required to attend. I also work with all of them on their grant proposals and their aims. The biggest problem that exists with young scientists writing their first proposals is that they think that they can solve the world's problems. You will solve nothing if you try to solve everything at the same time. They need to focus their research proposals and to propose to deliver the goods on a very narrow topic. Simplicity will always win. I also stress that their focus needs to be on their research passion and to think about their "t-shirt." I ask, "If you make a t-shirt that states a quick phrase that sums up your research, what will it say?" That is also one of my favorite questions to ask to young faculty members when they come for interviews. *What would you put on your t-shirt?* Communication and marketing *are* very important.

What are some other ways for marketing yourself and your institution? Every year we issue our annual Biomechanics Research Building newsletter. Some people would disagree with the amount of effort we put into it but for us, this endeavor is very important. We send it to everyone in our email database containing thousands of people. All these people receive our email that includes the annual newsletter. It's necessary. If it is important for Pittsburg; a huge city with long tradition and several extremely well-established research institutions, then it's triply important for us. Many people tend to think that Nebraska is all about cornfields and cows! We needed to change this perception and prejudice and help them to understand that, in Nebraska, we perform top notch biomechanics research.

2.9   *Characteristics of a successful grantsperson*

I want to close this chapter with what I consider the characteristics of a good grantsperson.

- *Makes a good first impression.* During a job interview, you have to dress nicely so that you will present the best picture of you. The first impression is always the most important impression. You need to create a good first impression with your grant too. This means no orthographical errors, no grammar errors, nice figures and pictures, bar graphs, and full justification.
- *Is well prepared.* Continuing on the previous example. After you deliver a good first impression, on the interview you need to show that you are well prepared. You will be asked simple questions on why you chose this particular organization. For example, I ask prospective PhD students who have approached me whether they have read my papers, which paper impressed them the most, and why specifically they wanted to come to my university. I want to examine if they are well prepared. So, how can you demonstrate that you are well prepared in your grants? You have to show that you have exhausted the literature and you cite the most important papers with respect to your question. You also have to provide preliminary data to show that you have already done some work on the project.
- *Is credible.* How can you be assessed in terms of your credibility? You can only establish credibility if you have a solid CV with excellent publications. If you had only one paper published in the past 10 years, then you will probably be rejected.
- *Delivers a clear message.* You should avoid talking uncontrollably in your interview. What should you say in an interview? The least you can say, the better. You should only say what is important. In terms of writing a grant, you should also go for simplicity. The more convoluted your proposal, the worse it will be. Write your proposal so that even people outside your field are able to understand it.
- *Provides supporting documentation.* You have to provide letters of support with your grant to enhance your application.
- *Has appropriate endorsements.* Your endorsements are the degrees that you have and the ones that you are currently working on from credible institutions.
- *Has something special to offer.* Why should you be hired? What is special about you? In terms of a grant, your special offer is *your idea*. Something fresh and novel.
- *Is persistent.* This is absolutely the most important characteristic of a successful grantsperson. In life, you will fail 10 times and win only once, and after that success you will fail another 10 times. This goes

for grants also. For all the grant proposals that I have had successfully funded, there are many more that were not funded. In life, persistence is the main quality you need to have in order to be successful. Here are some quotes to provide you with some additional motivation to be persistent. "I have not failed. I've just found 10,000 ways that won't work." Thomas A. Edison; "Only those who dare to fail greatly can ever achieve greatly." Robert F. Kennedy; "Success is measured by how high you bounce when you hit bottom." George S. Patton; "It is hard to fail, but it is worse never to have tried to succeed." Theodore Roosevelt; "Do not judge me by my successes, judge me by how many times I fell down and got back up again." Nelson Mandela

References

Bates, B.T., Stergiou, N. (1996). Performance accommodation to midsole hardness during running. *Journal of Human Movement Studies*, 31, 189–210.

Hardre, P.L., Beesley, A.D., Miller, R.L., Pace, T.M. (2011). Faculty motivation to do research: across disciplines in research-extensive universities. *Journal of the Professoriate*, 1(5), 35–69.

Lorenz, E.N. (1963). Deterministic nonperiodic flow. *Journal of the Atmospheric Sciences*, 20(2), 130–141.

Russell, S.W., Morrison, D.C. (2016). The Grant Application Writer's Workbook: Successful Proposals for Any Agency. Grant Writers' Seminars and Workshops (GWSW).

Smith, S.D. (2016). Factors that Motivate Faculty to Pursue External Funding at a 4-Year Public Institution of Higher Education. *Electronic Theses and Dissertations*. Paper 3011.

Wysocki, B. (2004). Research Advance: At Pitt, Scientists Decode the Secret of Getting Grants. *The Wall Street Journal*. Issue 28 June.

Young, J. (2003). *A Technique for Producing Ideas*. New York: McGraw-Hill Professional.

chapter three

Writing grant proposals

> All outstanding work, in art as well as in science,
> results from immense zeal applied to a great idea.
>
> **—Santiago Ramón y Cajal (1852–1934)**

3.1 Introduction

This chapter provides a comprehensive approach, with numerous examples and tips on how to write successful grant proposals. Emphasis is given on how to write grants for the National Institutes of Health (NIH). As one of my grant writing mentors, Dr. Jeff French once said, "if you know how to write grants for the NIH, you can write for any agency and funding source."

3.2 The basics

Whether you are applying for a federal grant or applying for a mini internal university grant, you will always have to have the following sections written. They may be called different things but they are pretty similar.

- *Specific Aims and hypotheses. What do you plan to do?* You will first need to include a paragraph that describes the Aims of your research study.
- *Background and significance. Why do you want to do this project?* Second, add a background paragraph that describes the previously published studies that are related to your Aims and hypotheses that shows the impact of your study.
- *Progress report/preliminary studies. What have you done so far?* Then you will have to provide preliminary studies, which will establish your credibility and prove your capability of executing that study.
- *Research plan. How do you plan to do what you propose?* Finally, you will have to describe the procedures of your research plan.

These sections need to be clearly described and outlined. Importantly, you live in a time that everyone is extremely busy,[1] and reviewers have very

---

[1] I recently asked my nephew how he was doing. He answered, "Uncle, you don't want to know!... I am *extremely busy!!*" He is ten...

limited patience because they have many other things to do. For that reason, you need to make sure that your proposal is one of those that is easy to read (even better, one that they will enjoy reading – more on that later). The basics for a well-written proposal are:

- *Well written, well organized.* Make sure the proposal is well written with no grammar or vocabulary mistakes. Always reach out for feedback from one of the scientists in your environment. Your paragraphs need to be organized in a consecutive order and be connected.
- *Accurate.* Always accurately cite the literature and refer to studies with genuine results. Reviewers are familiar with the literature and any inaccuracy will be recognized.
- *Good, clear visuals.* Present pictures in the methods section. Nowadays it is fairly easy to use your phone to take pictures of your experimental setup. In addition, present the results section using well-designed graphs. Do not use more than three lines if you want to present your results in a line graph. I personally prefer bar graphs and not line graphs, because line graphs can be confusing (by using multiple lines in the same graph that intersect).
- *Easy to read and understand.* Revise, rewrite until it is so. Use less words, not more. Think carefully about how to explain everything and use easy-to-read fonts (i.e. Times New Roman) and sufficient spacing.

3.2.1 *Specific Aims and hypotheses*

Special care needs to be given to this section of the proposal. It is truly the heart of the entire proposal. With all my students, postdocs, and young faculty members, we work extensively on a single page where the Aims will be clearly outlined. Only after we finish with this page we move forward with the rest of the proposal. As I mentioned in chapter one, proposals without hypotheses are viewed as "descriptive," that is, random searches for information. This is a cardinal error. If you don't have a research question, then you will just be gathering data. It will be very difficult to receive any funding without a specific research question. I personally ask my students to eliminate the word "describe" from their vocabulary if they want to become scientists. Here are some basics on how to write this section (see also chapter one).

Hypotheses should be…

…specific. The research needs to be specific, not broad.

…mechanistic. It should have a clear supporting rationale.

…tested by the specific Aims. The Aims and hypotheses should be intertwined.

...*not too numerous.* Even if you have promising hypotheses, you will not receive the funds if there are too many of them. It will come across as unrealistic and overambitious. You should have an agenda that allows you to finish the specific research study you are about to conduct.

...*well formulated.*

A poor hypothesis just states an expected result:

Variable A will correlate with variable B.

A good hypothesis is specific and tests for the mechanism through which a phenomenon occurs.

Variable A will positively correlate with variable B because...

By stating if it will be positive or negative and explaining why it correlates in that manner, you create specificity. How would you know to make that type of statement? From the literature and your preliminary data. A good hypothesis progressively solves a scientific mystery by choosing between various explanations. Here are some examples.

3.2.2   *Hypothesis examples*

Q1   HOW DOES THE PLATYPUS REPRODUCE?

either:
It lays eggs *or* by live birth *or* by mitosis.

Poor example of a hypothesis:
Platypus will frequently be seen with eggs.
Better example:
Platypus will frequently be seen with eggs because that is how they reproduce.
Still better example (an *if...then* statement):
If I watch a female platypus for a sufficient time after mating, then I will see an egg appear.
I have made it mechanistic.
Or for a hypothesis more related to Biomechanics...

Q2   WHAT IS THE EFFECT OF EARLY DEVELOPMENT ON BONE MINERAL DENSITY?

Poor example:
The bone mineral density (BMD) of children's bones is correlated with age.
This example lacks both specificity and the "because" factor.
Better example:
The BMD of children's bones increases with age because,

- *mineralization takes months.*
- *the remodeling rate declines with age.*
- *the average osteon has longer to mineralize.*

Practically, your *Overall Hypothesis* is "The BMD of children's bones increases with age." The word "increases" makes your hypothesis directional. Then you propose three mechanisms or three experiments that you will conduct to test this hypothesis. These experiments are independent from each other and each one will exclude a certain branching in your logical tree (chapter one). These three experiments are what we call our *Specific Aims* using the NIH language.

3.3   Writing grant proposals for the NIH

Now I shift gears and speak about how to write successful grants for the NIH. At the end it will be clear why with this information you will be able to write a successful grant for any agency.

3.3.1   NIH basics

The NIH is the primary agency in the United States that is responsible for biomedical and public health research. It was founded in the late 1870s and is now part of the United States Department of Health and Human Services. The majority of NIH facilities are located in Bethesda, Maryland. The NIH conducts its own research through its Intramural Program and provides major biomedical research funding to non-NIH research facilities through its Extramural Program. The NIH has an annual funding budget of over $30 billion (www.nih.gov/about-nih/what-we-do/budget#note). About 10% of the annual budget is directed towards intramural funds, for the NIH institutes to work on their own research. The NIH institutes have several laboratories and many brilliant professors and researchers dedicated to conducting research in their own specific scientific fields. In addition, some of that money is used for building supplies, equipment, and administration.

The NIH comprises 27 separate institutes and centers of different biomedical disciplines and has been responsible for many scientific accomplishments. The 2016 records show that the NIH have supported 149 Nobel Prize winners in the past. The NIH has also contributed significantly to the increase in life expectancy in the United States through their scientific and research contributions. An increase from 71 to 79 years of age was recorded between 1970 and 2010 (CDC, 2012). NIH scientific efforts have contributed to advances in healthcare combatting many pathologies such as heart disease, cancer, HIV/AIDS, and arthritis (NIH Health, 2016).

Several of the institutes have funded my research through the past years. Here are some examples. The National Institute of Biomedical Imaging and Bioengineering provided funding to host the American Society of Biomechanics meeting in Omaha at 2013. The Eunice Kennedy Shriver National Institute of Child Health and Human Development provided funding for a K25 developmental award and an R15 for a specific research project. More recently, the National Institute of General Medical Sciences provided with funding to develop the Center for Research in Human Movement Variability through the P20 mechanism.

3.3.2   Why has NIH been so successful?

They fund ideas, not institutions. They mostly care about the idea and not the institution within which the research will be conducted. An idea can come from anyone. If you have a good idea, you can receive NIH funds. You do not have to be at a prestigious university. Good ideas can spring from local researchers. For example, my NIH K25 grant came from the University of Nebraska at Omaha, a predominantly teaching university without even doctoral programs at that time. It was the first NIH K25 for our state.[2]

Researchers must compete (like entrepreneurs) for funding. Researchers must compete and perform their best. The NIH chooses the best application to be funded.

Scientific experts do the judging. NIH always use experts in each specific domain to review the application.

Universities receive funds only when their scientists submit successful applications. Scientists have to submit a successful application to receive the funds. Otherwise no funds will be obtained.

NIH program and review staff are separate. The Center for Scientific Review (CSR) is an independent center that has specific people in charge of recruiting reviewers for each grant proposal. The NIH Program Officers have no influence on the review board. This is extremely important so that the review board is not influenced by personal interest.

Scientists manage the peer review process. Scientists manage the review meeting as well as review the grant applications.

---

[2] People used to tell me that the NIH do not allocate funds based on the best applicants and best applications, but rather that they choose to fund the same people all the time or you have to belong to the "club." I was also told early on in my career that I would not be funded because I work at the University of Nebraska at Omaha. Do not believe any of this. I proved all these people wrong! The NIH system is extremely fair and the best I know. If you don't receive funds, this just suggests that you need to come up with a better idea and write a better grant. Just keep trying and persist.

3.3.3   NIH type of awards

There are many different types of NIH awards (https://grants.nih.gov/ grants/funding/ac_search_results.htm). I list several of them below, and these are the ones that I consider to be the most important.

- NIH Research Project Awards/Grants (R Series)
    - R03 – Small Grant Program. Small, starter grants. Pilot and feasibility studies.
    - R15 – Academic Research Enhancement Awards (AREA) for institutes without strong NIH histories. No preliminary data required.
    - R21 – exploratory/developmental grants. No preliminary data required.
    - R34 – Clinical Trial Planning Grant Program. This Grant is gaining momentum and several scientists are applying for it nowadays.
    - R01 – Research Project Grant Program.
- Program grants for large teams (P awards)
    - P20 – Research Program Projects and Centers.
- National Research Service Awards (NRSA)
    - F30/F31 – Predoctoral award.
    - F32 – Postdoctoral award.
- Career development grants (K series – Mentored Awards)
    - K25 – Mentored Quantitative Research Development Award.
    - K99/R00 – NIH Pathway to Independence Award.

As mentioned above, the NIH provides a tremendous amount of funding each year, distributed across several funding mechanisms. Table 3.1 shows the proportions of the total funding budget that NIH estimated it would allocate to the different mechanisms for the fiscal year 2017. Over 50% is allocated to research project grants (R awards).

3.3.3.1   The R01 award

The R01 award is the major funding goal for scientists who pursue research in health fields in the United States. This grant demonstrates independence for the scientist. It is the NIH's most commonly used grant mechanism. The award provides funding to support investigator-initiated research on a discrete, specified project. Investigator-initiated research, also known as *unsolicited research*, is research funded as a result of an investigator submitting a research grant application to NIH in the investigator's area of interest and competency. The NIH does not provide specific ideas but rather expect the scientist to investigate a specific problem within a

Table 3.1 Proposed Funding Allocation for Total NIH Funding
Budget for the Fiscal Year 2017.

Mechanism	Allocation (%)
Research project grants	54.9
Research centers	7.8
Intramural research	10.9
Research and development contracts	9.6
Research training	2.6
Research management and support	5.2
Facilities construction	0.5
Other research, superfund, Office of the Director	8.5

Source: HHS (2016).

broad field. That is why it is called "investigator-initiated research." There
is no specific dollar limit unless specified in the Funding Opportunity
Announcement (FOA). Advance permission is required if you are applying for $500,000 or more in any year. Nowadays they encourage scientists
to not exceed $300,000. An R01 is generally awarded for 3–5 years and is
utilized by all NIH Institutes and Centers.

You can have multiple R01 awards. As the R01 is renewable, you could
have it for your entire academic life. During renewal, however, you compete with other applications. Renewals are similar to when you initially
apply; the only difference is that you have a significant amount of data and
publications to strengthen your application. Early-stage investigator (ESI)
status is considered during the review. ESI is defined as an investigator
who has completed their terminal research degree or end of post-graduate
clinical training, whichever date is later, within the past 10 years and who
has not previously competed successfully as a principal investigator for a
substantial NIH independent research award. The FOA provides all the
information necessary about the requirements for the R01 (not including
font, structure, and style of the paper).

3.3.3.2   The R15 award
The R15 AREA supports small research projects in the biomedical and
behavioral sciences conducted by faculty and students in health professional schools and other academic institutions that have not been major
recipients of NIH research grant funds. The award Aims to strengthen
the institutional research environment and expose students to bio-
medical/behavioral research, but it is not specifically a training grant.
It requires expanded *Investigators* and *Resources* sections. The R15 has
its own Director, responsible for management of the AREA. The project
period is limited to 3 years. Direct costs are limited to $300,000 over the

entire project period. Multiple principal investigators (PIs) are allowed, if all are eligible. This grant is also renewable and preliminary data are not required but can be provided. This award also has unique review criteria as applications are scored on the likelihood of the project providing opportunities for students and bolstering the research environment of the applicant institution, as well as making an "important scientific contribution" to the field. Some specific review criteria that are unique to the R15 are the following:

- Significance – Will the project strengthen the research environment? Will the project expose students to research?
- PI – Does the PI have experience supervising students in research? The PI should include details of previous experience with student researchers.
- Approach – Can the project stimulate students' interests so they consider a biomedical/behavioral science career?
- Environment – Are well-qualified students available? Have previous students from the environment pursued biomedical/behavioral science careers? Are they likely to?
- Facilities – The facilities section should include details of the student pool and likely impact of the grant on the institution.

Because this award is one that my university is eligible for and I have been successful through this mechanism (as have several of my faculty), I have also included below some additional hints for prospective applicants.

- *R15s are research awards – not training grants. They support hands-on research experiences for students.* You should show plans to expose students to hands-on research but not detailed training plans as you would see in a fellowship or training grant application.
- *R15s must involve undergraduate AND/OR graduate student researchers.* The aspects of the project in which students will participate should be identified.
- *Postdocs are not considered students.* However, postdocs, technicians, or faculty collaborators may be included.
- *R15s are renewable and are considered career-sustaining awards.* For a renewal, you should evaluate your progress in the research and whether research experiences for students have been provided.
- *Facilities and other resources available should be appropriate for the proposed R15.* This section of the application should describe the student pool, the expected impact on the institution, special characteristics that make the institution appropriate for the R15, and institutional support. The focus here should be on the institution, not the PI's personal experience.

3.3.3.3 *The R03 award*

The R03 is for small grant applications, intended to provide limited funding for a short period of time to support investigator-initiated research. It supports different types of projects including pilot and feasibility studies; secondary analysis of existing data; small, self-contained research projects; the development of research methodology; and the development of new research technology. It is limited to 2 years of funding, with direct costs generally up to $50,000 per year. This grant is not renewable and the funding is meager for conducting major research studies. This is why its popularity has dropped in recent years. However, they are still quite useful grants to get your foot in the door, so to speak, and to help you conduct some additional pilot work for your R01 submission. They are utilized by more than half of the NIH Institutes and Centers.

3.3.3.4 *The R21 award*

The R21 is for exploratory/developmental grant applications. The R21 is similar to the R03 but provides more funds. It is intended to support the early stages of project development in investigator-initiated research. It is limited to up to 2 years of funding and the combined budget for direct costs for the 2-year project period cannot exceed $275,000. No more than $200,000 may be requested in a single year. Preliminary data are generally not required, but may be included if available. It is utilized by most NIH Institutes and Centers.

3.3.3.5 *The Ruth L. Kirschstein NRSA*

The Ruth L. Kirschstein NRSA program offers two types of grants:

- *Training grants (Ts).* Awards used to support predoctoral and/or postdoctoral research training activities. Applied for by institutions.
- *Fellowships (Fs).* Awards for pre- and postdoctoral students. Applied for by individuals.

The NRSA fellowships are awarded to pre- and postdoctoral fellows who are working under faculty mentors. The training can be delivered at either a local or a foreign institution, where the field of study is directed to basic and clinical research as long as it fits the mission of the NIH institutions. All applicants must meet the following core review criteria in order to be considered for any of the Fellowship awards.

- Applicant's capabilities – Reviewers will assess applicants' academic records and training (Grade Point Average, Graduate Record Examination scores, and transcripts), publications (published manuscripts), and academic presentations (national and international conferences presentations).

- Sponsors, collaborators, and consultants – Reviewers also assess the mentors' previous achievements and how that will affect the candidate. Criteria include the mentors' previous awards and grants.
- Research training plan – This will indicate whether the candidate is likely to receive comprehensive training in all areas required in order for them to be successful.
- Training potential – The potential of the candidate and their mentor.
- Institutional environment and commitment to training – The reviewers evaluate the commitment to the award and training through letters of support provided by the mentors. Mentors have to express that they will be committed to training the candidate. The mentors' previous accomplishments with other PhDs or postdocs are crucial to this section.
- Training in the Responsible Conduct of Research – Potential fellows are assessed through their previous classes in research conduct. Attaining the appropriate research skills is a necessity for fellows before applying for F awards.

The Predoctoral Fellowships, F30 and F31, are awarded to MD/PhD and PhD students, respectively. The F30 (since 1989) supports up to 6 years of combined MD/PhD training. The F31 (since 1974) supports up to 5 years of PhD (or equivalent) training/dissertation research. This is a fantastic award that two of my students have received. It sets their career very nicely in terms of support for their PhD years and strengthens immensely their CVs for future endeavors. There is also a dedicated Diversity F31 intended to support individuals from populations that are traditionally underrepresented in clinical research careers.

The F32 (since 1974) supports up to 3 years of postdoctoral research training. The 2017 (NIH grants, 2017) stipends range from approximately $43,700 for a new postdoc to $57,500 for one with 7 or more years of experience. It is a good idea for PhD students to start applying for the F32 award before applying for a postdoc. It is advisable to start working with the future postdoc mentor on applying for a F32 during the final year of the PhD. The budget is not limited to researcher stipends. Additional expenses (e.g. travel, equipment) can also be included. Over the last 20 years, the number of predoctoral fellowships awarded has increased while the postdoctoral fellowships have been decreasing.

3.3.3.6   *The Career Development Awards (Ks)*

The Career Development Programs (Ks) provide protected time for individuals to further develop their research expertise. There are K awards for postdocs such as the Pathway to independence award (K99/R00), and for early career faculty such as the mentored research scientific developmental award (K01), the mentored clinical scientific research career development award (K08), the mentored patient-oriented research career development award (K23), and the mentored quantitative research career development award (K25). There are also K awards for Midcareer faculty such as the Independent scientist award (K02) and the Midcareer investigator award in patient-oriented research (K24), and even for senior faculty such as the Senior Research Scientist Award (K05). The success rates of K awards vary. I had the pleasure of supervising a postdoc (Dr. Leslie Decker) who received a K99/R00 award, and I personally received a K25 early in my career. Both had tremendous impact on our personal careers. In Figures 3.1 and 3.2, I have provided data of the success rates of the two that I have personal experience in; the K25 and the K99/R00.

I should mention here that some K awards such as the K08, K23, and K24 require a clinical degree (PT, MD, etc.). Previous NIH PIs may be ineligible for these awards. Usually a previous PI on an R03 or R21 grant is acceptable, but not if you had a K99/R00. A PI on a previous or current R01 or subproject PI on a P01 is not eligible for a K award.

The K awards are awarded for up to 5 years. The K99 phase of the K99/R00 is a minimum of 12 months but generally no more than 2 years. Mentored awards require full-time effort, defined as at least 9 person months or 75% of their time is to be allocated to research and the rest on other career development related activities. Regarding budget, salaries are capped between $75,000 and legislatively designated mandated cap, while research/development costs are generally $25,000–$50,000

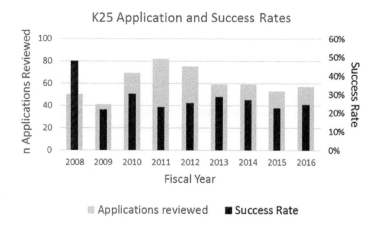

Figure 3.1 Approximately 25% of the K25 applications reviewed in 2016 were successful. This has been fairly consistent since 2009.

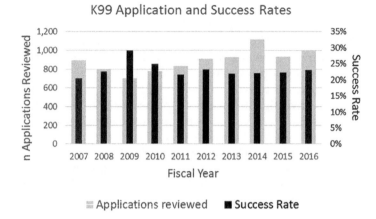

K99 Application and Success Rates

▬ Applications reviewed   ■ Success Rate

Figure 3.2 The K99 success rate has been fairly consistent over the past 10 years. In 2016, about 23% of the applications reviewed were successful. You can see that there are far more K99 than K25 proposals submitted.

(i.e. supplies, equipment, technical personnel, travel to research meetings or training, tuition/fees, computational services). Normally the indirect cost is set by the institution but, interestingly, the K awards' indirect cost is set and unchangeable, at 8%. Thus, several institutions do not encourage their employees to apply for the K awards. This is why you need to make sure that you have the support of your Chair.

The K99/R00 is the brainchild of the previous NIH director, Elias A. Zerhouni. This award was introduced to overcome the problem that many postdocs encounter: they keep gaining experience through consecutive postdoc appointments without achieving a faculty position. The K99 award was introduced so that postdocs can receive 2 years of funded postdoc training, but also 3 years of R-based funding at the institution who will hire them as faculty members. Thus, the recipient becomes highly desirable because of this R-based support, which leads to bright career opportunities. Applicants must have had no more than 4 years of postdoctoral research experience (previously 5 years). In order to transition from the K99 to R00, applicants must finish a minimum of 1 year of the K99 postdoc award.

The K awards also have additional review criteria that deal with the quality of the Candidate, the Career Development Plan, the Research Plan, the Mentor(s), Consultant(s), Collaborator(s), and the Environment and Institutional Commitment to the Candidate.

In summary, grant mechanisms for training and career development are available for all stages in your career. In Figure 3.3, I have provided a

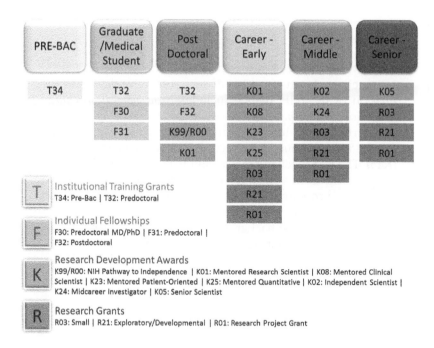

PRE-BAC	Graduate /Medical Student	Post Doctoral	Career - Early	Career - Middle	Career - Senior
T34	T32	T32	K01	K02	K05
	F30	F32	K08	K24	R03
	F31	K99/R00	K23	R03	R21
		K01	K25	R21	R01
			R03	R01	
			R21		
			R01		

T Institutional Training Grants
T34: Pre-Bac | T32: Predoctoral

F Individual Fellowships
F30: Predoctoral MD/PhD | F31: Predoctoral | F32: Postdoctoral

K Research Development Awards
K99/R00: NIH Pathway to Independence | K01: Mentored Research Scientist | K08: Mentored Clinical Scientist | K23: Mentored Patient-Oriented | K25: Mentored Quantitative | K02: Independent Scientist | K24: Midcareer Investigator | K05: Senior Scientist

R Research Grants
R03: Small | R21: Exploratory/Developmental | R01: Research Project Grant

Figure 3.3 Your career through grant proposals.

Research Training and Career Development Timeline to assist scientists, especially, in terms of the proper timing of application for each award.

3.3.4 The K25 grant – an example

In this section, I will demonstrate how I use the guidelines of a specific grant mechanism to actually write the grant. As I mentioned in the beginning of this chapter, and in the previous one, this is what I do with any grant I write. Here, I will be using the NIH guide for the mentored quantitative research career development award (K25) program announcement (PA) alongside the K25 grant proposal that I wrote and got funded, back in 2002. Some of the particulars have changed since then (it is essential that anyone applying for this, or any other grant, downloads the most current PA); however, the way of tackling it remains the same. The PA that I used was the PA-02-127. The K25 grant, at the time, was supported by 17 NIH Institutes including the National Institute of Child Health and Human Development (NICHD), to whom I applied.

The first thing that I always do when I write a grant is to read the PA many times, and underline or highlight words that are extremely important for the application (see Vignette 3.1).

VIGNETTE 3.1

"A particular area of research is often invigorated by *novel* perspectives. In an effort to advance research relevant to the mission of the NIH (which includes *basic biomedical, clinical biomedical, bioengineering, bioimaging,* and *behavioral research*), the participating institutes and centers solicit applications for the *mentored quantitative research career development award* (K25). The K25 mechanism is meant to attract to NIH-relevant research those investigators whose *quantitative* science and engineering research *has thus far not been focused primarily* on questions of health and disease. Examples of *quantitative* scientific and technical backgrounds considered appropriate for this award include, but are not limited to: *mathematics, statistics, economics, computer science, imaging science, informatics, physics, chemistry, and engineering.*"

All of the italicized words that are mentioned in the PA purpose statement are extremely important keywords that need to be addressed and followed while writing the grant. See more below.

I then start writing the different sections of the grant. Note: all Vignettes in 3.3.4 are directly taken from the text of my K25 award.

3.3.4.1   Section 1. Introduction to revised application
This section is only included when the proposal is a resubmission.

VIGNETTE 3.2

"I would like to thank the reviewers of the Initial Review Group for their *insightful* comments. In this Introduction, I will specifically address each of the concerns raised by the reviewers in the order that they were discussed in the Summary Statement. The requested changes have also been designated in italicized text in the revised career development award application."

Always make sure you include a *thank you note* in your introduction (see Vignette 3.2.; here I thank them for their "insightful" comments).[3] In your resubmission (and also your original application) you want to

---

[3] The word "insightful" is also important. They are not simply comments. They are "insightful" comments.

show your best side. Words such as *disagree* should not be included in any circumstance.

The Introduction to Revised Application section should list *all* of the concerns raised by the reviewers alongside their solutions. It took me a long time to understand the importance of addressing *ALL* of the reviewers' concerns, with a significant cost, unfortunately! Previously, this section had a three-page limit; now it is only one page. I used to include each concern on a separate line but this is no longer possible with the reduced page limits. Now I tend to include short summary statements that bring multiple comments together. Something like "Reviewers 1 and 3 had some concerns with recruiting." I also include a table that clearly presents the previous reviewers' scores for each criterion (see Table 3.2). Remember, *the reviewers are very busy people.* It is your job to make sure that all the comments and scores are mentioned clearly in your first section, because the reviewers will not have time to go back and review your previously submitted application.

Nowadays, you only have the opportunity to revise the grant once. You can also submit the revised version as a new application, however, and this essentially means that you can reapply as many times as you want. Your decision as to whether to revise or not should depend on the language of the reviewers. If the reviewers raise issues with the research question, experimental design, and the idea itself, or if the reviewers display a distinct lack of enthusiasm, then it may be better not to revise and resubmit. On the other hand, if the reviewers appear enthusiastic and the issues that were addressed are minor and related to logistics then you should revise and resubmit. In order to have a better sense of the reviewers' enthusiasm through their comments, you should call on someone with experience in the process.[4]

Table 3.2 Example Table to Use in the Introduction to Revised Application with the Reviewer's Scores.

	Criterion			
	Environment	Investigator	Significance	Approach
Reviewer 1	Score	Score	Score	Score
Reviewer 2	Score	Score	Score	Score
Reviewer 3	Score	Score	Score	Score

---

[4] Lack of mentorship is a "death penalty" in science. I still contact my PhD mentor, Dr. Bates, and ask for his advice to this day. I did my PhD over 20 years ago. I personally mentor several students and faculty members specifically for help with grant proposals, many of whom are not even current or previous students of mine. You will always need a mentor, and that is why before you change environments you must make sure that there will be a mentor there to guide you.

Now, let us move to examine how I addressed specific concerns.

VIGNETTE 3.3

"1.A. Rationale for specific coursework/absence of educational objectives gained by the coursework.

Reviewers 1 and 2 raised a concern regarding the rationale for specific coursework. Specifically, Reviewer 1 mentioned that although the focused areas for coursework seem very reasonable, there were no educational objectives or definition of skills to be gained by the coursework. To address this concern, I have included the educational objectives for each of the proposed courses."

I addressed these comments by including all educational objectives for each course (see Vignette 3.3). I did *exactly* what the reviewers wanted.

VIGNETTE 3.4

1.B. Addition of a motor control expert as a consultant or mentor to strengthen the application.

Reviewers 2 and 3 suggested the addition of a motor control expert as either a consultant or a mentor to strengthen the application. Such an expert can advise me regarding neural and postural control mechanisms. In addition, the expert can also advise on the usage of the linear measures acquired. Subsequently, I have added the expertise of ...., Ph.D. for the University of .... as a consultant. He will guide my analysis of the linear measures of postural sway, as well as he will advise me regarding neural and postural control mechanisms. Dr. .... is a motor control specialist that has received several R01 grants from the NIH to investigate how multisensory inputs interact in the control of human upright stance, and how children use sensory information to control balance. Through the duration of the award, I will travel at least once a year to his laboratory and I will present my research progress to him for continuous critique and feedback. I will also interact with him electronically and via phone to receive additional guidance and direction.

I addressed the comments by adding a consultant who specialized in motor control (see Vignette 3.4). Again I did *exactly* what the reviewers wanted.

VIGNETTE 3.5

1.C. The inclusion of a population with "benign congenital hypotonia (BCH)" may be problematic.

Reviewer 1 had a concern that the inclusion of infants with BCH might be somewhat problematic because this is a fairly heterogeneous population. The reviewer suggested that a CNS imaging criterion such as "periventricular leukomalacia" would create a less heterogeneous study group. However, I would like to mention that the methodology I wish to study is not a test for verifying or determining the etiology of a movement disorder, but rather a test that will differentiate among a group of infants to better describe, treat, and evaluate their postural control. I chose to examine a group of infants who are symptomatically homogeneous; infants who will all have hypotonia. Infants who have periventricular leukomalacia would likely be heterogenous in their symptoms although homogeneous in the etiology of their motor disorder, with some infants having severe symptoms of cerebral palsy and others having mild tone disorders or decreased movement. Rather than choose a group that is homogeneous in their etiology, I want to study a group that is homogeneous symptomatically. This will allow differentiation among problems of postural control without other confounding variables. I do plan to look at infants with other diagnoses in the future, but in the present application I would like to focus on infants with benign congenital hypotonia. Additional rationale for this choice has been included in the application.

Here I used a different approach (see Vignette 3.5). I disagreed without mentioning the word disagree. I did not change the methods as the reviewer had requested, but the rationale I provided in this section (and added to the application itself) was the change towards meeting the reviewers' comments that was needed. Always try to do at least a small portion of what the reviewers are asking – never do nothing.

VIGNETTE 3.6

1.D. Addition of motion analysis for kinematic measures and addition of electromyography (EMG) measures.

Reviewer 2 suggested the addition of kinematic measures during sitting to understand the strategies used to obtain the center of pressure (COP) measures. Consequently, I added the kinematic measures of trunk angle and pelvic angle to the dependent variables. Previous studies (included in the Background section) that have examined EMG in infants have utilized perturbation paradigms, either via platform perturbation or a moving visual surround. These studies have measured the variables of temporal order of muscle activation, latency to muscle onset from perturbation, or co-activation related to the perturbation. Since there is no perturbation, measurement of EMG will be difficult to quantify.

For this comment (see Vignette 3.6), I added the kinematics measures but not the EMG measures. It would have been immensely difficult with the infants to use EMG. However, again I did "something" instead of nothing, and at least added the kinematics. Thus, I met the reviewers half way.

3.3.4.2 *Section 2. The candidate*

This is a section specific for mentored awards but also helps everybody to understand the mechanics of writing successful grants. Throughout this section, I used language taken directly from the PA to create all the subheadings. I also used all the keywords that I highlighted in the PA in my writing (see Vignette 3.1). The first part was on academic training (see Vignettes 3.7–3.10).

VIGNETTE 3.7

"My training in biomechanics built a *foundation* for developing the *skills* needed to perform *independent quantitative biomedical research*."... "I obtained my PhD in Biomechanics from the University of Oregon in 1995, *with a strong quantitative and technical background that can be applied to diverse areas of research*."

The italicized words/sentences are taken directly from the PA. I presented my quantitative background utilizing similar wording. Remember that the reviewers will first read the PA to familiarize themselves with the mechanism, before judging the grant proposal. If they then recognize the required attributes within the grant proposal, it will have a higher chance of being funded. This merely points the reviewer to them!

VIGNETTE 3.8

"My undergraduate studies were conducted in Thessaloniki, Greece, and led to a BS in Exercise Science (1989). My curriculum included instruction in human anatomy and physiology, biochemistry, exercise physiology, physics of human movement, ergonomics and motor development. During these studies, I developed an interest in biomechanics."

I described all of my quantitative courses from my undergraduate degree and avoided the irrelevant ones (see Vignette 3.1 and 3.8).

VIGNETTE 3.9

"This interest in biomechanics led me to pursue graduate work at the University of Nebraska at Omaha where I was awarded a graduate assistantship. My graduate studies in this university led to an MS in Exercise Science with an emphasis in biomechanics (1991). This degree included instruction in research methods, statistics, motor learning, advanced exercise physiology and biomechanics. *I also continued building my technical and quantitative abilities by taking courses in mathematics and engineering such as calculus, differential equations, ergonomics, engineering statics and dynamics, and strength of materials.*"[5]

Here I tried to demonstrate my enthusiasm and dedication during my graduate studies, by pointing out the engineering courses that I took that

---

[5] This is also an example of how I was building my academic career, taking advantage of every opportunity I possibly could to gain knowledge. Ergonomics was an optional course, but I took it. When I was a student, if there was an interesting lecture across campus, I would attend. This is the time where you will develop your arsenal. This is the time where you will build your knowledge; your foundation; your "bank account" to be able to make your "withdrawals" at a later time.

were not a part of my curriculum (see Vignette 3.9).[6] The language always points directly to the PA and helps portray me as a quantitative scientist (see Vignette 3.1).

VIGNETTE 3.10

"Therefore, I decided to continue my graduate work at the University of Oregon where I was awarded a research assistantship. In this program, I took concentrations of courses in *biomechanics, motor control, and computer science.* I also enhanced my classical mechanics background with *advanced graduate physics courses.* However, during my doctoral education I mostly focused on nonlinear dynamics. I became very interested in this domain and thus, I pursued further quantitative training in mathematics by *taking graduate level instruction in matrix algebra, advanced differential equations, discrete dynamical systems,* and especially *mathematical chaos theory.*"

I got a minor in mathematics during my PhD, in addition to the other quantitative courses (see Vignette 3.10).[7] The reviewers are slowly persuaded that I have a solid quantitative background that makes me not only eligible but also a strong candidate for this award (see Vignette 3.1).

The second part of the Candidate section was on Research Training (see Vignettes 3.11–3.17).

VIGNETTE 3.11

"From the beginning of my graduate education in biomechanics, I have received *intense* training in statistical and research methods."

---

[6] During my graduate education, some of my friends mocked me because I was studying and working hard all the time, taking all these extra courses that I wasn't obligated to take. The K25 was the payback for all of my nights of hard work and dedication. The K25 allowed me to apply for, and obtain, more federal grants and, ultimately, to build my entire career. Keep working hard and, like the mythical hero Heracles, when having to choose between a pleasant and easy life or a difficult but glorious life, choose the latter.

[7] Another senior doctoral student (Dr. Howard Davis) and I were the only doctoral students who had a minor in mathematics. Howard managed it in addition to having his wife, Bizzi, and four children at home. He should be an inspiration to all. He is always mine.

The language is extremely important (see Vignette 3.11); here the reviewers will almost "feel" the intensity of the training that I received in statistics! I actually undertook eight courses in statistics. So, it was truly intense!

VIGNETTE 3.12

"Thus, I lack the experience to work with children, including specific *clinical populations*. It is a *major goal of this career development award to gain experience* in working with children and *clinical* pediatric subject populations."

You have to mention your strengths and weaknesses. Here I mentioned my lack of experience in clinical research because that was the primary criterion for the K25 award (see Vignette 3.12). The K25 award supports a transition from quantitative research to research with clinical populations. I described a lack of experience in clinical research but also my strong, independent experience in quantitative research. In addition, I keep "sprinkling" the application with the language from the PA (see highlighted words and Vignette 3.1).

VIGNETTE 3.13

"I have conducted *biomedical research* since August 1989, when I started my graduate education in biomechanics. As a doctoral research assistant at the University of Oregon, my primary advisor was Dr. Barry Bates. I shared his interest in the study of human movement variability and coordination and how they relate with *clinical problems* during gait. During this time, I participated in *biomedical research* projects that examined: movement variability within-subjects and between-subjects, the effect of footwear on performance variability, and the relationship between lower extremity joint coordination and injuries during locomotion. In these projects I used several types of *biomedical research analysis* such as signal processing, inverse dynamics to quantify joint moments and powers, and regression analysis. Several research papers resulted from this work."

As I present my previous research and publications, I continue to demonstrate that I am a strong quantitative scientist and, thus, an excellent candidate (see Vignette 3.13). I explain all of my quantitative work and finish with citations of my own publications to clearly establish my credibility.[8]

VIGNETTE 3.14

"Recently, I started collaborating with clinicians (..., PT,..., MD, one of the mentors of this award, and ...., PT) from the University of Nebraska Medical Center, on issues related with sitting postural development in infants. We used nonlinear methods to examine longitudinally the development of sitting postural control in five infants with typical development.[my references] We evaluated postural sway to understand sitting independence, which is one of the first motor milestones achieved by a child. Our results showed increased regularity, as a more stable sitting posture evolves, indicating a more periodic strategy of maintaining sitting postural control. We also found that early in development, infants restrict their degrees of freedom. However, as sitting independence emerged, we observed a possible release of the degrees of freedom. This preliminary work[my references] provided me with an exposure to child motor development research. To expand these interests, I would benefit tremendously from a period of training as described in this career development award."

In this Vignette 3.14, I explain the work I have done in the motor development field. This is in order to demonstrate commitment and preliminary work in the field. No preliminary work was required for this award but I am a strong believer that to have preliminary work always helps, and strengthens your credibility.

VIGNETTE 3.15

"My potential to conduct research as an independent investigator is indicated by the large number of my scientific publications. *Specifically, I have authored or coauthored 23 peer-reviewed journal articles, 7 book chapters and 70 conference abstracts. I have also 5 more peer-reviewed journal articles in press and 15 under review.*"

---

[8] Before you apply for this grant or any grant, you should prove that you are credible by demonstrating your publications. Pave your way with publications!!!

In the Candidate section, I created subsections to specifically address every single goal of the PA. Meticulously wrote about every single one of them. In this subsection (see Vignette 3.15), I address the *Candidate Potential to Develop into an Independent Investigator.* Even though I was teaching three courses a semester till the time that I received this K25, I was able to publish more than 20 papers and several book chapters in a few years. I always say to my students: "You cannot outsmart anyone, but you can outwork everybody."

VIGNETTE 3.16

"I have a strong background in biomedical research working with healthy young adults. During my career I have applied numerous types of engineering and advanced mathematical analyses to biological signals. *As my research progressed from biomechanical to clinical biomedical,* I realized that *I need additional training to improve my abilities to work with different types of clinical populations.* Thus, my immediate career *objective* is *to obtain the educational background and the experience needed to successfully perform research* with children and other clinical pediatric subject populations."

I first describe my previous (strong) background in quantitative biomedical research with healthy young adults. Then, I introduce my lack of knowledge with a clinical population for which I need the additional training that the K25 will support (see Vignette 3.16). The reviewers will not score you high because you need the training, but because you are an excellent candidate to receive this training, and will be highly successful in the future if you do so. In addition, I never stop using the language from the PA, strategically placing words throughout the grant proposal.

VIGNETTE 3.17

"My research training will be guided by two respected mentors, ... MD, and ... PhD. Dr. ... MD is a professor in Pediatrics at the University of ... and the Associate Director of the .... Dr. ... PhD is a professor of psychology and biology at the University of Nebraska at Omaha."

This was a mentored award so I needed to have a mentor (see Vignette 3.1 and Vignette 3.17). Since this was a clinically oriented application, I needed to have as a mentor an excellent clinician scientist who was also a pediatrician. I was able to identify Dr. ... MD from our Medical Center. Usually one mentor is sufficient, but I added a second because a mentor should be available in the environment in which the research will be done. Dr. ... PhD is a professor at UNO. In addition, Dr. ... MD did not have R01 funding, while Dr. ... PhD did. Dr. ... MD is a pediatrician. Dr. ... PhD has tremendous experience in developmental psychology.[9] It is very important to be strategic in every aspect of your application. In addition to these two mentors, I added three consultants: a motor control specialist, because my research was going to be on postural control of developing infants; a mathematician, because I was going to use nonlinear analysis; and a physical therapist, as the ultimate goal of this research was going to be improved rehabilitation. By having such a team, I was able to cover all my bases and demonstrate to the reviewers that I can collaborate. None of these mentors and consultants received funding from this grant because the budget was minute ($50,000). This demonstrates how wonderful these people were. However, I would like to stress that it is important to allocate funds to the mentors and consultants in your grants, because that will demonstrate their commitment to the reviewers.

3.3.4.3   Section 3. The research plan/strategy

This section is present in all NIH grants and, as mentioned above (Section 3.2), exists in some form in all grants. The very first section is the Specific Aims (see Vignettes 3.18–3.20). The NIH Specific Aims is just one page and, as I mentioned in chapter two, I work extensively on this page before I move any further. I prefer to have three paragraphs before I write an overall hypothesis and the associated Aims (see Section 3.2.1). In these paragraphs, I write the following:

- Paragraph 1 is the problem.
- Paragraph 2 is what has been done so far and why this is inadequate.
- Paragraph 3 is what I have done so far for this problem that has led me to the overall hypothesis.

Then I list the overall hypothesis and the Aims (see Section 3.2.1). I close with one more paragraph on the impact of my proposal. As a reviewer, I read the Aims even before reading the abstract. It is the most important

---

[9] Dr. ... PhD actually works in developmental psychology with marmosets. I never mentioned the marmosets as my research was with human subjects. However, he was the only scientist in my institution with an R01. So, I had to use what was available to me.

section. If the Aims are interesting, then I start reading the grant in detail. If not, I start looking for weaknesses.

VIGNETTE 3.18

"Specific Aim #1: To determine the reliability of the nonlinear tools, including intra-session and inter-session reliability."

This was the first Aim of my K25 (see Vignette 3.18). It is important to choose your words carefully when you write your Aims. "Determine" indicates a strong sense of identifying problems and finding solutions. Verbs such as "describe," "evaluate," and "assess" should not be used in the Aims.

VIGNETTE 3.19

"H1.1. We hypothesize that the nonlinear tools of dimensionality, complexity, and stability will have high intra-session and inter-session reliability when used to analyze the COP time series during sitting.

H1.2. We hypothesize that the known linear measures such as the length of the COP path will not have high intra-session and inter-session reliability when used to analyze the COP time series during sitting."

Two hypotheses were presented for Specific Aim #1 (see Vignette 3.19). You will notice that the second hypothesis is the opposite of the first but for different outcome measures. These demonstrate that I know my data and have a sense of how the results will come out. When you cannot put forward a directional hypothesis, always use an "If... then" statement.

VIGNETTE 3.20

"Specific Aim #2: To investigate whether increasing ability for postural control of typical infants affects nonlinear measures during sitting."

"Investigate" is a magnificent verb because it conveys your *in-depth search for solutions* as an investigator; another Sherlock Holmes, as we spoke in chapter one (see Vignette 3.20). Presenting your ideas in a powerful fashion will certainly affect the reviewers' opinions. The excellent presentation of a good idea will give the edge over other good ideas in a highly competitive funding arena. However, you cannot turn a bad idea to a good one with an excellent presentation. Never forget this.

After I have finalized my Aims page, I start writing the rest of the grant. I organize it using the following subsections: (a) Significance, (b) Innovation, and (c) Approach. These subsections point the reviewer directly to where the NIH evaluation criteria are located in my grant. Here are also some hints on how to write the rest of your grant:

Hint 1: It is extremely important to have well-designed graphics. I used to pay an artist to create proper graphics for me (Figure 3.4). However, nowadays you have the capability to create phenomenal graphs using different types of software. Graphics can explain what you plan to do, or your experimental set-up, much better than lengthy text. They also break up the text providing relief for the eyes of the reviewers. I recommend that you consider including graphics for your theoretical model, your logical tree, and your data collection process. Always provide a clear timeline graph at the end of your proposal (Figure 3.5).

Hint 2: Start your Approach section with your preliminary data, organized by Aim. Then describe your proposed methods, again organized by Aims. Include in your Approach: a power analysis, a sample size justification, and a section on anticipated problems and how you are going to address them. Never forget to clearly explain your recruiting procedures and your inclusion/exclusion criteria.

Hint 3: Organize the entire grant using a numbering system. For example:

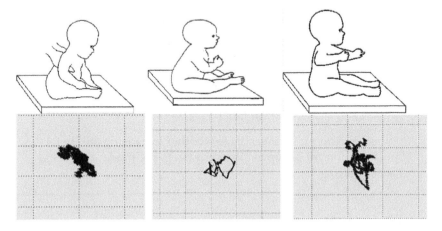

Figure 3.4 It is extremely important to use well-designed graphics. In this figure, the babies were drawn by an artist. The pictures demonstrate the postures of the babies vividly.

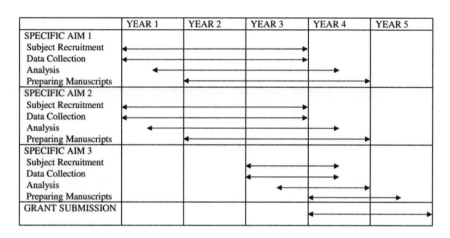

Figure 3.5 A sample timeline.

1. RESEARCH STRATEGY
1.A. SIGNIFICANCE
1.A.1. Specific problem statements
1.A.1.a. Trans-tibial amputees have markedly decreased sensory input.
1.A.1.b. The coupling between the prosthesis and the residual limb is not rigid.
1.A.1.c. Amputees' output (movement) and input (sensation) are degraded.

And so on...

This system allows you to present everything in an organized fashion and when you want to refer to previous sections, you can refer them by this numbering system.

Hint 4. Regarding formatting, I prefer Times New Roman as a font. I always use full justification to make the paragraph neat and professional-looking. I indicate references with numbers using superscripts because I can save space. I use bars on the side of the page to indicate where the changes are when I prepare a revised application.

3.3.5 Understanding the NIH grant application submission process

Identify a NIH Program Officer that can answer questions about your grant. You may have to go through the list of available Program Officers at the NIH Institute webpage or you can ask your colleagues about someone who is helpful. This person is your most important contact. *Contact them early and often!* Most of them are extremely helpful. I contacted my Program Officer during the development of my K25 grant. She was exceptional. She read my entire grant and corrected it like a reviewer, and practically wrote the Specific Aims page with me. During application preparation, Program Officers can provide technical assistance and advice. For example, I was working with scientists from Arizona State University on an R21. The PI wanted me to be a co-PI, but I didn't feel comfortable as I would not be available for the data collection process and felt that that would affect the grant negatively. I suggested I should be a named consultant on the grant instead. For reassurance, we contacted the Program Officer, who supported the solution I had suggested. Several Program Officers attend the meeting where the applications are reviewed. They cannot speak during these meetings; only observe and take notes. After the Study Section meeting, it is the Program Officer who provides you with the feedback necessary to address the comments that arose during the meeting. After your award is made, the Program Officer remains your main point of contact if you have any questions about the grant or need to make any changes to the budget, personnel, etc.

3.3.5.1 Additional hints for a successful submission process

- Get started well in advance. Crafting a strong application will take more time than you anticipate, especially if this is your first NIH application. Start early enough that you'll have time to solicit feedback and revise the application before the deadline.
- Identify the appropriate funding announcement. Read the general application guide in addition to the PA. Get information from your institution. Gather your questions and get answers from trusted individuals.
- The NIH website has a specific section that provides all the information needed about grant and funding requirements (www.nih.gov/grants-funding).
- Use the NIH database RePORTER (https://projectreporter.nih.gov/reporter.cfm). The database RePORTER provides a record of all the previously funded NIH grants. The entire abstract of each funded grant is available to the public. You can use this database to identify the institutes related to your topic of interest. You can identify ideas that have not been published in yet but received funding to be explored. This allows you to change your idea if you find a similar one already funded. Note: graduate students who are interested in pursuing their PhD or postdoc with a specific professor can search for the funded grants of that specific scientist, and find out when the funds will end.
- Make sure you know your deadlines so that you can submit your application in good time (see also chapter two). You also have to make sure that your proposal is being reviewed by the appropriate reviewers (i.e. Study Section). If your research is directed towards musculoskeletal biomechanics, your proposal should not

be reviewed by a bunch of psychologists. Furthermore, don't forget to check the "Status of Your Application" in eRA Commons. eRA Commons is the online interface where grant applicants, grantees and federal staff at NIH, and grantor agencies can access and share administrative information relating to research grants.

- You submit your grant to Grants.gov. If no errors are found by the automatic checking systems, it is placed in a queue. When the grant is retrieved by an agency, further checks are made against the agency's business rules. You must check the status of your application in eRA Commons as this is where any errors and warnings that you need to attend to will be displayed. Errors will halt the application process. Warnings can be addressed or left at your discretion. You have two business days to carefully check your assembled grant in eRA Commons.

3.3.6   *Understanding the NIH grant application review process*

After you submit the application to the NIH, the application goes through the following process:

1. CSR – reassigns your application to a Study Section.
2. Study Section – reviews the application for scientific merit, then sends it to the actual Institute (note, there are a lot of Study Sections).
3. Institute – evaluates the application for relevance.
4. Advisory councils and boards – recommend the final action: fund/ do not fund the application
5. Institute Director – makes the final decision as to whether the application will receive the funding or not.
6. Fund allocation – you receive the money if you have won the grant.
7. Research conducted!

The Gateway for NIH Grant Applications is the CSR.

- Receives all NIH applications.
- Refers them to NIH Institutes and Centers and to scientific review groups (Study Sections).
- Reviews about 70% of all NIH applications for scientific merit: the other 30% of applications do not even fit the criteria. The application is declined without review.

In 2013c, the Center for Scientific Research (CSR) received 84,000 applications, 236 Scientific Review Officers recruited 17,000 reviewers. They went through 1,500 review meetings to finalize the funded applications. The existence of this center is a major reason for the success of the NIH. They make sure that NIH grant applications receive fair, independent, expert, and timely reviews, free from inappropriate influences, so that the NIH can fund the most promising research.

3.3.6.1   *The cover letter*

The cover letter that you include with your application is vital for this process, as it serves a number of important purposes.

- *Suggest Institute/Center assignment.* You can suggest the specific institute to review your grant application.
- *Suggest review assignment.* Applicants can suggest a specific Study Section to review their grant proposal.
- *Identify individuals with a potential conflict.* Candidates can exclude specific reviewers that could potentially harm the proposal due to personal bias. A detailed explanation must be included, for example, a statement explaining a difference in theoretical perspective.
- *Identify areas of expertise needed to evaluate the application.* Even if the application is likely to be reviewed by experts in the appropriate field (e.g. biomechanics), you can recommend that it is evaluated by reviewers that are knowledgeable in a more specific area of the field (e.g. animal biomechanics).
- *Discuss any special situations.* Applicants can discuss any additional aspects relevant to the project, for example, the need to recruit specific pathological populations.

It is NOT appropriate to use the cover letter to suggest specific reviewers. Instead of mentioning specific reviewers by name, indicate a specific field of study and they will pick appropriate reviewers to the best of their knowledge. The following cover letter (Vignette 3.21) was used to highlight a special review situation to avoid it being sent to the wrong institute and describes what the research project is focused on in order to get knowledgeable reviewers. It is advisable to recommend two institutes instead of one because this will increase the chance of receiving funding.

VIGNETTE 3.21   Sample cover letter

Please assign this APPLICATION "TITLE" (PA-XXXXXXXX) to the following:

Institutes/Centers
  National Institute of Aging
  National Institute of Neurological Disorders and Stroke

> Scientific Review Group
> Musculoskeletal Rehabilitation Sciences Study
> Section – MRS
>
> Please do not assign this application to the following:
>
> Scientific Review Group
> Biophysics of Neural Systems Study Section – BPNS
>
> This study focuses on a new in vivo model for investigating … (A FEW WORDS ON WHAT YOU ARE DOING, TO GET APPROPRIATE REVIEWERS) …, but not … (A FEW WORDS ON WHAT YOU ARE NOT DOING, TO AVOID GETTING INAPPROPRIATE REVIEWERS).

3.3.6.2   The Study Section

Funding is based on two levels of review. The first level of review (90% of the decision) is the scientific review group (Study Section), where the application is being reviewed by your peers. The second level of review (10% of the decision) is the NIH advisory council, made up of intramural and extramural scientists and administrators. The advisory council make the final decision based on availability of funds, also factoring in legislative mandates. The council assesses the quality of reviews and can decide if the review is applicable to the institution or not. They also decide on the budget and may or may not support the amount requested in the application. The council will not alter the scientific evaluation or score.[10]

The Study Section includes about 25 reviewers from different institutions (university, government, industry scientists) that are both "regular" and "ad hoc"; one regular member is Chair, and a Scientific Review Administrator (SRA) is NIH's overseer. Usually the Study Section reviews from 40 to 140 grant proposals in each session. Other NIH administrators

---

[10] At the VA, an advisory type of council meeting is conducted just hours after the Study Section, whereas the NIH council meeting occurs after several months. During the council meeting, the chair, administrators, and Scientific Research Officer (SRO) gather around with the reviewed grants. During one VA advisory council meeting I chaired, two reviewers gave a score of 1 for a particular grant proposal, while the third reviewer provided a score of 5 without any justification. The reviewers couldn't come up with a consensus and the scores remained the same. As the Chair, I felt that the applicant had received a score that was not reflecting the quality of the proposal, maybe due to some bias from the third reviewer. I suggested the inclusion of a different reviewer whose score, if closer to 1, could result in the grant being funded. The administrators accepted my suggestion, which provided the applicant a better chance of being funded.

are usually present. A few NIH administrators will be present by phone. Each proposal is assigned to a primary reviewer, a secondary, and usually a tertiary reviewer, and sometimes two to three "readers," who do not write a full review. Sometimes additional readers are assigned to help ease the process. Each reviewer has about 10 reviews to write and several proposals to read. Each proposal has more than 20 pages. Applicants must take this into account and make the proposal as clear as possible with no mistakes. Everyone is free to discuss/comment. In addition, everyone scores every proposal.

Usually the NIH hires temporary reviewers to review grant proposals. Temporary reviewers count for two thirds of the entire review board. The SRA, who heads the Study Section, decides which reviewers are most suitable to review an application and whether there are (or ever have been) conflicts of interest between reviewers and applicants, such as collaborations, coauthorship on research papers, or other interactions. The average scores of the three last meetings of the Study Section are taken to even out different scoring tendencies. Some reviewers are harsher than others, and taking an average makes the likelihood of receiving funding more consistent across meetings. During the Study Section, the SRA and Chair are considered ethics watchdogs. They will call on and judge the reviewers who did not step out of the room when they had the need to due to any conflict of interest. In addition, they will judge any reviewers that provided inappropriate comments that may have influenced other reviewers' opinions. No discussion about any of the material presented during the Study Section is allowed to take place outside the meeting. Everything must be discussed as a group within the meetings. The environment is extremely professional and all the reviewers must follow the same professionalism. *Note: Differences between NIH, National Science Foundation (NSF), and the Department of Veterans Affairs (VA)*. Based on my experiences, at the NSF the Program Officer is usually the SRA and the Chair at the same time. The Program Officer is the one responsible for making sure that the proposal receives a fair review at the NSF. The VA is slightly different to the NSF as the Program Officer is the SRA but there is an independent Chair.

The reviewers in the Study Section are not blinded to the applicants. Blinding is impossible because qualifications must be assessed.[11] Reviewers leave the room for the discussion if they work at the applicant's institution, or if

---

[11] Reviewers can find out anything about the applicants – they can search for everything about you in social media and the internet in general. They may be told not to do so... but they may still do it... or may just become "friends" of yours on Facebook. I am not sure if this is some form of bias – I guess it depends on what you call Facebook friends! Anyway, all this can create issues or bias toward the applicant. Be careful what you include on social media and the internet. Stay away from politics and any other topic that may harm your grant application (or any job application).

they are otherwise close to the applicant. A reviewer is considered close to the applicant if they have any type of work relationship. Friendship is not considered a conflict if the two individuals did not share any previous work relationship.

Applications are scored from 1 (highest) to 9 (lowest) (Table 3.3). Scores of 5 or lower are normally streamlined. For a score of "3" ("excellent") or above, the application must be considered very strong with negligible or only minor weaknesses. These should be easily addressable, and not substantially lessen the impact of the proposed work. Scores of 4–6 (medium impact) indicate moderate weaknesses, that is, weaknesses that lessen impact.

3.3.6.3 The meeting of the Study Section – what happens behind closed doors

Streamlining immediately shelves 50% of the proposals. Practically, at the start of the meeting, the reviewers provide a list of the proposals they reviewed that fell in the bottom half. If the assigned reviewers agree and

Table 3.3 Guidance for Scoring Used by Reviewers.

Impact	Score	Descriptor	Additional guidance
High	1	Exceptional	Exceptionally strong with essentially no weaknesses
	2	Outstanding	Extremely strong with negligible weaknesses
	3	Excellent	Very strong with only some minor weaknesses
Medium	4	Very good	Strong but with numerous minor weaknesses
	5	Good	Strong but with at least one moderate weakness
	6	Satisfactory	Some strengths but also some moderate weaknesses
Low	7	Fair	Some strengths but with at least one major weakness
	8	Marginal	A few strengths and a few major weaknesses
	9	Poor	Very few strengths and numerous major weaknesses

Definitions:
Minor weakness: Easily addressable; does not substantially reduce impact.
Moderate weakness: Reduces impact.
Major weakness: Severely limits impact.

there are no objections, these proposals will be triaged. These proposals will not be discussed, although the reviews will be sent to the applicant. Anyone in the meeting can object with no argument necessary. Note that a review with a score of "5" (considered "good") will not usually make it to the Study Section meeting and will not receive an overall score and a percentile. This indicates that a *very good* proposal is required even to be discussed by a Study Section. Many reviewers feel the need to provide a good score, even if the proposal is poor. That should not happen. A fair score should always be presented, even if it means giving a score of 8 or 9.

Each proposal is usually discussed for a duration of 20–30 min. After the reviews are discussed by everyone present (except the Program Officers), the members of the Study Section rescore the proposals. Reviewers cannot score outside the range of the three reviewers' previously stated scores. For example, if the three reviewers scored 2–4 the other members of the Study Section must provide a score between the 2 and 4. Any score outside this range must be well justified. After reviewing all the applications, the mean score of all Study Section members is calculated then multiplied by 100. There is a major difference between the final score and the percentile, where the percentile is calculated by the formula: $100 * \frac{(\text{Rank} - 0.5)}{N}$, where N is the total number of applications in the set.[12]

Finally, the budget and ethics are discussed after scoring.

In a recent NIH Study Section meeting I participated in, we started the reviewing process with proposals from the young investigators who had applied for an R01 grant. The R01 applications were grouped together and only 50% were discussed (ten proposals). Next we discussed the R01 proposals from established investigators. These were also grouped together and 50% of them were discussed (11 proposals). Finally, all of the other applications were grouped together (R21, R15, and R03). There were 25 proposals in this category. Seven were R15 and only one R03. The rest were R21s. Only 50% were discussed (12 proposals).

3.3.7 Main review criteria

The applicant needs to apply and address these criteria in the proposal.

Overall Impact. The *Overall Impact* is the assessment of the likelihood of the project exerting a sustained, powerful influence on the research field(s) involved. This is a novel section that has been introduced in the past 10 years. Several individuals confuse this with the Significance section (Vignette 3.22). This section will strengthen the applicants' proposal if it shows the project may have a major overall impact. Hint: You must

---

[12] I remember we once received a score of 20 on an R21 proposal. Even though this is a good score, the percentile was not high enough to be approved and receive funding.

create an Overall Impact section and explicitly state the words "Overall Impact" to attract the reviewers' attention.

Significance. Is the research study significant in terms of tackling an important health problem? Funding will be directed towards proposals that address major clinical problems (e.g. cancer) instead of pathologies that affect only small populations (e.g. rare diseases). Does the project address an important problem or a critical barrier to progress in the field? If the Aims of the project are achieved, how will scientific knowledge, technical capability, and/or clinical practice be improved? How will successful completion of the Aims change the concepts, methods, technologies, treatments, services, or preventative interventions that drive this field?

VIGNETTE 3.22 What is the difference between impact and significance?

Impact. Will the research exert a sustained, powerful influence on the research field?
Significance. Does the research address an important problem or a critical barrier to progress in the field?

Investigator(s). Are the applicants dependable and credible? Can they be relied upon to conduct this research? Are the PIs, collaborators, and other researchers well suited to the project? If there are ESIs or New Investigators (NIs), do they have appropriate experience and training? A NI is an NIH research grant applicant who has not yet competed successfully for a substantial, competing NIH research grant (i.e. R01). An ESI is a new investigator who has completed his or her terminal research degree or medical residency – whichever date is later – within the past 10 years and has not yet competed successfully for a substantial, competing NIH research grant. If established, have they demonstrated an ongoing record of accomplishments that have advanced their field(s)? If the project is collaborative or multi-PI, do the investigators have complementary and integrated expertise; are their leadership approach, governance, and organizational structure appropriate for the project?

Innovation. Is it a novel proposal? Does the application challenge or seek to shift current research or clinical practice paradigms by utilizing novel theoretical concepts, approaches or methodologies, instrumentation, or interventions? Are the concepts, approaches or methodologies, instrumentation, or interventions novel to one field of research or novel in a broad sense? Is there a refinement, improvement, or new application of theoretical concepts, approaches or methodologies, instrumentation, or interventions proposed?

Approach. In addition to a well-planned experiment, the methods section needs to have preliminary data (for most funding mechanisms), statistics, recruitment plans, and sample size calculations that are appropriate and relevant to the study. Are the overall strategy, methodology, and analyses well reasoned and appropriate to accomplish the specific Aims of the project? Are potential problems, alternative strategies, and benchmarks for success presented? If the project is in the early stages of development, will the strategy establish feasibility and will particularly risky aspects be managed?

Environment. The applicant should have the appropriate space and equipment to facilitate the research study.

The reviewers use these criteria to write their critiques. These critiques are placed on a specific template and are written in the form of bullet points (strengths and weaknesses) or, if necessary, short narratives. The goal of such critiques is to write evaluative statements and to discourage summarizing the application. The critique template contains a total of 18 boxes. Reviewers should provide text for only those criteria that are applicable. The SRA at the NIH writes the abstract of the summary statement for the proposals that have been discussed at the Study Section.[13]

1. Overall impact	7. Resubmission	13. Biohazards
2. Significance	8. Renewal	14. Budget and Period of Support
3. Investigator(s)	9. Revision	15. Select Agents
4. Innovation	10. Protection of Human Subjects	16. Applications from Foreign Organization
5. Approach	11. Inclusion of Women, Minorities, and Children	17. Resource Sharing Plan
6. Environment	12. Vertebrate Animals	18. Additional Comments to Applicant

These write-ups are included in the Summary Statement that you eventually receive back from the NIH. In general, the Summary Statement will have:

- *Study Section roster.* The roster will both include the reviewers who are always part of the grant review and additional novel reviewers.
- *Scores* for each review criterion.
- *Reviewers' critiques.* Significance, approach, innovation, investigator's qualifications, research environment, overall evaluation.
- *Administrative notes,* if any, for example, biohazards, no inclusion of minorities.

[13] In contrast, at the NSF and the VA the first reviewer is assigned to write the abstract of the summary statement for each proposal.

If your application is discussed, you also will receive:

- *Overall impact/priority score and percentile ranking.* The percentile is essential in this process.
- *Summary of the discussion.* The summary of discussion is written by the SRA.[14]
- *Budget recommendations.*

When you receive the Summary Statement you need to carefully review the critiques and make a decision as to whether the proposal is worth resubmitting or not. Many applicants do not know what to do after receiving the Summary Statement. Advice from more experienced scientists should be sought. Make sure you *carefully analyze the critiques.* What was uniformly disliked? What should be changed vs. re-explained? What additional data could be provided? Are there words of encouragement embedded in the criticisms? Are significant strengths mentioned? Do the comments suggest above average enthusiasm? It is advisable to throw the grant into the garbage can if it receives very bad review scores. *Always revise if the chance of successfully addressing the comments seems good.* A previous student of mine sent me two summary statements and asked for feedback. I recommended her to resubmit the proposal that received the worse score because the critiques were more constructive and the issues were fixable. She received funding. Even though the other proposal had a better score, it did not have such a good chance of receiving funding. It is extremely important to be able to address the reviewers' comments. Begin with addressing the reviewers' criticisms in the Introduction to the Revised Application. Always try to meet the reviewers half way, be gracious, respond positively, and never use negative vocabulary (e.g. disagree).

3.3.8   Exercise: A mini proposal review for the NIH grant titled "The Six Million Dollar Corpse," originally devised by Dr. Thomas Buchanan from the University of Delaware and respectfully revised by Dr. Nick Stergiou from the University of Nebraska at Omaha

The numbered references listed below for the model grant are not related to the text of the book.

Abstract. Crash dummies have been employed for simulating traumatic injuries in humans since the 1920s [1]. Recent advances in crash

---

[14] In other institutions such as the NSF and the VA, it is the job of the primary reviewer to write the summary of the discussion.

dummy technology have given us dummies with realistic constitutive properties for skin [2,3], bones [4–6], and even internal organs like liver [7], stomach [8], and brain tissues [9,10]. However, to date no crash dummies have included any structures that resemble the human neuromuscular system. This is a significant problem because muscles are the key structures for stabilizing the joints [12–20]. The goal of this project is to design a Muscle Activated Crash (MAC) dummy that, in addition to the constitutive properties of passive tissues found in other models [2–10], will have realistic muscles and reflexes. The key to MAC's uniqueness will be his artificial muscles made from polyacrylonitrile fibers [21]. These fibers will be used because they exhibit Hill-type force–velocity relationships [22] and have similar passive constitutive properties to normal muscles [cf 23 and 24]. To make MAC realistic, 16 muscles that span the neck, spine, shoulders, elbows, wrists, hips, knees, and ankles will be included. In addition, MAC will have a nervous system that will provide realistic reflexive feedback to the muscles so that they can be used to stabilize the joints. Data for the basic constitutive properties of MAC will be taken from previous crash dummy studies [25–29]. Reflexive muscle activations will be recorded from EMGs during simulated driving accidents in instrumented stuntmen and stuntwomen. MAC will be compared to data from a generic crash dummy: the Deafferanted Unmuscularated Mannequin Body (DUMB). In a series of crash tests, we believe it will become apparent that MAC is superior to DUMB in modeling traumatic injuries.

Critique based on review outline for NIH grant
Significance

- People get killed or seriously injured in car crashes every year. These injuries constitute a major component of national health-care costs.
- Crash dummies are widely used for studying traumatic injuries. But current ones cannot simulate the neuromuscular responses.

SCORE: 3

Innovation

- Perceives a need in the field and attempts to fill it in a unique way. The lack of soft tissue responses in current crash dummies is a serious shortcoming.
- In principle, adding such responses could represent an important innovation.
- The use of polyacrylonitrile fibers is an interesting and novel means of modeling active as well as passive tissue properties.

- While novel, the feasibility of the project is low (see approach)
- Even though the proposal is innovative, it received a low score due to the approach section that influenced it.[15]

SCORE: 4

Investigators

- Written by a reputable investigator who received his PhD in Biomechanics from the University of Oregon in 1995. He is currently the Professor of Biomechanics and Director of the Center for Research in Human Movement Variability at the University of Nebraska Omaha.
- Although he has a strong background in biomechanics, he has no publications in this area.
- Needs additional collaborators: statistics, chemical engineering.

SCORE: 5

Approach

- Strengths:
  - Based on solid principles of biomechanics and neuromuscular physiology.
  - Attempts to validate model with real data.
- Weaknesses:
  - Cute language (MAC and DUMB) is strained and doesn't help. *[This wouldn't be articulated in the review.]*
  - Hypotheses are not clearly articulated and are not testable – no possible statistics.
  - Lacks preliminary data.
  - It would be outrageously expensive and so technically difficult that the likelihood of success is low. It would take forever to get so many muscles to work properly. Overly ambitious.
- More weaknesses
  - The approach is naïve. Most traumatic injuries occur so quickly that muscles do not have time to be activated.
  - Polyacrylonitrile fibers resemble real muscle, but are about 100 times slower, making them useless for this study.
  - Instrumenting stuntmen (and stuntwomen) in auto accidents? This would not receive human review board approval.

---

[15] If the proposal is innovative but cannot be realistically conducted, then the Innovation score will be negatively affected.

SCORE: 8

Environment

- As stated, the project would be strengthened by the addition of a Chemical Engineer knowledgeable in polyacrylonitrile fibers.
- It is unclear whether or not the investigators have the facilities to perform crash tests on conventional and polyacrylonitrile-equipped dummies.

SCORE: 5

Overall Impact

- This is a surprising naïve proposal from highly regarded expert in biomechanics.
- It will have no impact in the field due to its low likelihood of success.
- This proposal would be recommended to be streamlined.

OVERALL SCORE = 7

3.4   Top Ten common reviewer concerns

These concerns are important for any grant you may write.

1. There are no clear hypotheses, nor well-defined goals.
   - Provide a focused hypothesis and clear objectives.
   - Describe the importance and relevance of your problem.
   - Be clear on how your project will move the field forward.
2. The Specific Aims do not test the Hypothesis, or the Specific Aims depend on results from previous Aims.
   - The best proposals are those with independent specific Aims that address your hypothesis using different approaches.
3. The proposal is not mechanistic, or not scientifically relevant.
   - Do not propose correlative studies, propose strong associations.
   - Do not propose general observations, propose specific manipulations.
4. The application is not appropriate for the grant mechanism.
   - An R21 is not an R01. A Career Development Award (K) is not a Research Project Grant (R). The opposite is true also.
   - If you are applying for an R21, do not treat it as an R01. You will not have the time nor the resources to complete it.
5. The proposal is overly ambitious.
   - Set realistic goals for the budget and project period you propose.

6. The proposal lacks preliminary data.
   - Include preliminary data for all Aims.
   - Use preliminary data to show knowledge of methods and data analyses.
   - But propose to do more than just confirm preliminary results.
7. It is not clear that the investigator can do the proposed experiments.
   - Don't propose what you can't do.
   - Include collaborators and consultants on your project.
   - Describe the value of datasets and experimental models.
8. The background section is missing key publications and experimental findings.
   - Thoroughly describe the literature, especially controversies, but....
     - Support your views and ideas.
   - Be sure you have found key references.
   - Make sure you provide a thorough description of the literature because reviewers are highly educated in these areas and will most likely be aware of all the relevant findings.
9. Experimental details, alternative approaches, or interpretation of data are inadequately described.
   - Don't assume the reviewers know the methods.
   - Provide alternative experimental methods you might employ should you encounter problems.
   - Show the reviewers that you have thought about your research plan.
   - Include pictures – a picture is better than 1,000 words. Nowadays we have easy access to cameras in our smart phones. Take advantage of that and use it to your benefit.
10. The proposal is not relevant to the mission of the institute.
    - Make your application fit the mission of a particular institute.
    - Don't try to force your application on an inappropriate institute.

3.5 A ten-step plan for losers – originally devised by Dr. Thomas Buchanan from the University of Delaware and respectfully revised by Dr. Nick Stergiou from the University of Nebraska at Omaha

These steps are applicable to any grant you may write!

1. Don't Include Hypotheses!
   In reality, the secret to "doing research" is to go into the lab, measure a bunch of things, and see what looks good. Just write in your

proposal that if you get the grant you will try to do things using Plan A. If that doesn't work, you'll think of a Plan B, etc....until you get things working. This is the classical "shotgun" approach, and it is especially popular among engineers. In fact, this is what separates engineers from scientists (who are confined by the so-called "scientific method").

2. Be Ambitious!

   A good proposal is one that demonstrates to the reviewers that you have lots of ideas, so write them all down. Don't worry if you are proposing enough work for 10 or 15 years – the reviewers will tell you which ideas they want you to pursue.

3. Cool Tools Rule!

   If you have developed a model or an engineering method that nobody else has, write a proposal that uses the model in as many ways as possible. These uses do not have to be related to a common problem or even to each other – reviewers will know good science when then see it! Show them how cool your method is and do not worry about trendy phrases like "biological relevancy."

4. For Clinicians: Don't Worry About Engineers!

   Submit your proposal to the NIH, not the NSF. There are no engineers at NIH. Only use very simple engineering whenever necessary – about the level of a freshman physics course – because addressing clinical problems is key. Do not reference state-of-the-art engineering approaches or else the reviewers will not be able to follow you. Besides, what are the chances that they would ask someone like a famous engineer like Dr. Scott Delp to review your proposal?

5. Statistics Are for Anal-Retentive People!

   When you write about data analysis, just say something like "I will do statistics on the data." The reviewers will understand what you mean. They all know that you will feed your numbers into a computer and look for the best "p" values, so don't mess with the details.

6. Remember: Hypotheses Are Simply Your Good Ideas!

   If you feel compelled to formulate hypotheses (despite #1 above), make sure that they are grand and glorious. They should not be specific enough to be testable. Furthermore, once they are described in the opening section, you should never refer to them again. Your goal (beyond getting funded) is to do science, not to test hypotheses.

7. Use Creative Writing!

   The introduction of fictional characters into your proposal who explain things to the reviewer is highly effective. This adds the needed human element and helps to avoid all those passive sentences.

8. "Preliminary Work" Is Not Cost Effective!

The granting agency wants you to do some of the work before they give you the money. Don't let them trick you! They are just trying to save costs. If you do substantial previous work, they will fund you for less time. Economically, it is far better to have a poorly developed "previous results" section than to solve all of the hard problems without being paid for it. Just stress in your proposal that you are a professional and you will be able to solve any problem that arises.

9. Be as Technical as Possible!

Try to impress the reviewers with your knowledge of math or engineering. For example, if you are describing the 3D geometry of the surface of the knee, refer to it as "a manifold in n-space." Another great strategy is not to assume your coordinate systems are orthogonal. Remember, if the reviewers have trouble understanding your proposal and are left scratching their heads, they can only conclude that you are smarter than they are.

10. Researchers Are Not Bean Counters!

The "budget sheets" are boring parts of every proposal where you are asked how much money you want. Enter big numbers here. Don't mess with a lot of prose justifying why you need a 16-processor supercomputer. We all know that you need it because it will be cool and those who get grants get cool things! Never mind that you won't use it for much beyond word processing. Hey, you are going to need something to write that next proposal on a few years from now!

References

CDC. (2012). CDC National Vital Statistics Reports. 60(4).

HHS. (2016, February 16). FY 2017 Budget in Brief – NIH. Retrieved September 9, 2017, from www.hhs.gov/about/budget/fy2017/budget-in-brief/nih/index.html

NIH. (2016, March 17). Our Health. Retrieved September 9, 2017, from www.nih.gov/about-nih/what-we-do/impact-nih-research/our-health

NIH. (2017, March 06). Budget. Retrieved September 9, 2017, from www.nih.gov/about-nih/what-we-do/budget#note

chapter four

Writing manuscripts

> If you wish to be a writer, write.
>
> **—Epictetus (AD 55–135)**

4.1 Introduction

One of the most fundamental aspects of academic life is writing scientific manuscripts. Thus, the scope of this chapter is to assist novice investigators in writing scientific manuscripts and identify critical writing mistakes. These skills are also important for anyone who wishes to write in science.

4.2 The scientific manuscript

Even if you may have read thousands of scientific manuscripts, writing one is completely different. A lot of people are fearful of writing scientific manuscripts which creates issues in their academic career, since published manuscripts are the main evidence of a scientist's work in academia. You will be measured on your success through your published manuscripts.

The scientific manuscript has the following components: title, abstract, introduction, methods, results, and discussion. Below I present how you can write each one of these components effectively.

4.2.1 Title

What's a good title? The title needs to be not too generic and not too grandiose and should reflect the major finding of your study. You must think very carefully about your title as it will be targeted directly by bibliographic search engines. When someone searches the literature using tools, such as PubMed or Web of Science, keywords are typically sought within titles and abstracts, or just within titles. If the title is too generic and unspecific, it is less likely to be found. If it is bland and non-compelling, it is less likely to be read. How many times have you just read the title and if you found it interesting, then you started reading the rest of the manuscript? Many authors underestimate the value of their titles, and this is a very big mistake. Here are some example titles:

- *Bad title*: "The effect of caffeine on blood pressure." This is an example of a poor title since it is very generic and does not describe the major findings of the study.
- *Better title*: "Caffeine affects blood pressure" OR "Caffeine does not affect blood pressure." This title is better than the previous one because it is specific and provides a vivid outcome with either a positive or a negative finding.
- *An even better title*: "Caffeine increases blood pressure." This title is even better because it is directional (i.e. increases) and therefore more specifically describes the major finding of the study.

4.2.2 Abstract

After the title, the first thing that the potential reader will peruse is the abstract. The abstract is one of the most crucial parts of the manuscript. When writing, many people leave the abstract until last. This is fine, but it should not mean that the abstract is an afterthought and not worth considerable attention. Again remember that is usually searchable and commonly targeted by search engines. Many times is the only part of your manuscript that will be read besides your title.

A lot of writers struggle with the first sentence of the abstract. My advice is to start directly with your research questions, hypotheses, or purposes, then describe your method in a few brief statements. Including key quantitative results within the abstract provides concrete information for those subscribing to abstracting services. Present the key findings only, and do not use generic statements. Also, ensure that results are directional, for example, a "significant decrease/increase." End with the answers to the questions or, in the case of a Technical Note, by emphasizing the utility and novelty of your design or approach.

4.2.3 Introduction

As with the abstract, many writers struggle with the start of the introduction. Aristotle said that "beginning is half of the entire task" and he was probably right. So how do you start with your introduction? First, you have to justify the need for the study. The key is to arouse interest. You have to imagine the readers sitting in front of you and you need to get them excited by providing a compelling rationale for the study. If you can't answer the question *"So what?"* you have a problem. Ask yourself what you consider to be the most interesting facts about the topic. Arrange your thoughts (and the paragraphs that are based on them) so that they have a logical flow. Remember Strong Inference and your logical tree (chapter one). Each paragraph should follow on from the previous one so that you are gently guiding the reader though from the knowledge gap (which provides the rationale for performing the study) to how you plan to bridge it[1]. Make sure you use references to support every declaration you make.

In general, I prefer that you include only the work that is most relevant to your study – do not burden the reader with a comprehensive literature search, no matter how knowledgeable you think it makes you appear. Don't bore the reader with endless prose. In other words, the introduction should be brief, and in most cases, need not contain more than four paragraphs, or two pages using double spacing and a reasonable sized font (e.g. 11–12 points).

Length is often dictated by the journal. Many journals impose restrictions although some have no limits and you can practically write a novel and it will still be published! However, as I said I prefer the introduction to be brief. For an original article, focus on the primary biological and/or clinical question(s) or hypothesis(es) you are addressing. In general, simple is better. Short sentences are easier to digest than long ones that try to talk about too many ideas at once. It is the same with paragraphs. *Is this sentence absolutely necessary?* If not, eliminate it!

Have a *purpose statement* right near the end of your introduction; "The purpose of this study is …" If you have done a good job with your introduction, the reader shouldn't even need to read the purpose statement. It should be implicitly obvious through your logical flow of evidence and arguments leading up to it. Try it! Give your introduction to a colleague but cover up the end of the introduction. If they can guess what the purpose of your study is, your introduction is well constructed. Importantly, end the introduction with your *hypotheses*.

We already covered construction of hypotheses in chapter two but briefly remember that your hypothesis is what you believe. For example, "Gender has an effect on the way we walk." The alternative hypothesis is "Gender has no effect on the way we walk." Based on your preliminary data and the previous literature make sure that your hypothesis is directional: "Specifically, females will walk faster than males." Note: In many cases, your hypotheses may not be directional, for example when your preliminary data cannot help you to state a clear directional hypothesis. In that case, you can use an "if…then" statement. Here is an example: "If attention to non-motor tasks affects locomotion, then we would expect that variability will be altered in subjects that have a greater attentional load, in comparison with those that do not."

4.2.3.1 Additional hints for the introduction
Hint 1: Make sure your introduction provides the theoretical underpinning for the variables you will measure, so that they don't come as a surprise in the methods (or results) section.

---

[1] When I was a graduate student, I used to record myself explaining the introduction. This was a major help.

Hint 2: Define important words, and avoid abbreviations. If you are using specialist terms that are important to your study but uncommon, make sure you define them in the introduction before you start using them. It is better to avoid abbreviations and acronyms. It disrupts the flow if the reader has to look back to hunt for their definitions.

Hint 3: We are living in a time when information is easily accessible and available to us, and people don't have time to read everything. If you don't write simply and compellingly, no one will read your article. Write so it can be understood not only by your mentor, but also by someone with a Bachelor's degree in Philosophy, or General Studies, or Physics or Nursing.

Hint 4: Make sure your introduction is consistent with your methods. As mentioned above, the final paragraph of the introduction should explicitly state the questions, hypotheses, or purposes you intend to explore. These questions should match the statistical analysis you will propose in the methods section. If you have a new statistical analysis (i.e. an additional independent variable) that is introduced in the methods section that was not mentioned in the introduction, the paper will be denied. That is because it was not justified in the introduction.

Hint 5: Never forget strong inference.

4.2.4   Methods

In the methods section, you need to justify everything you did. Show that you have thought of everything, and that you are meticulous. The key? Attention to detail. You can organize your methods into the following subsections:

- Subjects (sample description: anthropometrics, consent procedures, demographics, inclusion and exclusion criteria, sample size justification, etc.)
  - Make sure you include all selection criteria. Note, this information enables the reader to determine whether your results are generalizable to the population that they are interested in. In the methods section, it is also vital to state that any protocol for human or animal subjects was approved according to the relevant laws and regulations of your country and institution.
- Experimental protocol (parameters measured and their selection)
- Data collection (Instrumentation, measurement techniques)
- Data analysis (procedures, special algorithms)
- Statistical analysis (factors, independent variables)

4.2.4.1   Additional hints for the methods

Hint 1: You need to include sufficient detail such that it would be possible for another scientist to replicate your study.

Hint 2: Make sure you include a paragraph detailing your statistical analysis and relate your statistical analysis to your hypotheses. The statistical analysis should *perfectly match* the hypotheses stated in the introduction. Never introduce new independent variables in the methods section.

Hint 3: Use figures! You cannot underestimate the power of pictures. I actually like pictures in the methods that clearly show the experimental setup (always make sure to take photographs and/or videos of your experiments so you can present them later on as figures in your paper, or its supplementary material).

4.2.5   Results

Your results need to be specific and unclouded. Your message will be clear if you begin each paragraph with a statement of a key result (parenthetically referring to data figures and tables) based on the framework of the hypotheses posed in the introduction. Follow the same order as that in which the hypotheses are presented in the introduction and outlined in the statistical analysis of the methods section. The most common statement that reviewers dislike is "The results for Variable X are presented in Table 4.1." This sentence is a waste of space because the table caption will be saying exactly the same thing. Instead, state what has happened to the variable (e.g. significant decrease or increase or no change) then put the table or figure number in a parenthesis to direct the reader to the numbers qualifying your statement.

Another important part of the results is the inclusion of figures (and tables) to describe your findings. Make sure that they clearly convey your major results. I actually recommend that you create your figures before you even start writing your manuscript. Figures in a manuscript should tell the story without forcing the reader to read the text. Yes, they'll be missing out if they don't read the whole, exciting yarn, but a lot of people prefer to save the time and jump right to the pictures! So start by drafting the figures and then write around them. The results section is all about figures. Slightly expand the captions for the figures to include the major result (again within the context of your questions, and complementary to lead sentences in each paragraph of the results section).

4.2.5.1   Additional hints for the results

Hint 1: The results section should contain only *your* results, and not cite those of others.

Hint 2: Avoid description of methods or interpretation of the results. These should be left for the methods and discussion sections, respectively.

Hint 3: One of the benefits of creating tables is it provides others with the ability to try to replicate your results. Be extremely careful. Ensure everything is accurate because once the article is published, it will be published forever. Always triple check.

4.2.6   Discussion

The discussion section is nearly always the most difficult to write. It is an interpretation of the data you have displayed in the results section. Be humble and don't make elaborate, unsupported statements[2]. You need to organize your discussion based on your previous hypotheses as described in your introduction, methods, and results, and *in the same order*. They need to match throughout the sections of the manuscript. You will also need to compare your results with other studies and discuss those for each hypothesis. Each statement should contain a key argument for or against your approach or answering explicitly posed questions. If the reader considers only the first sentence of each paragraph, he or she should not miss any important information. Furthermore, the flow of that information should logically lead them to the same conclusions that you have made. In terms of organization, you can use the following layout.

- *How the results relate to the theory?* Separate paragraph for each hypothesis. Is it supported by your results? Answer the question you posed in the introduction. Discuss it with respect to the literature. Do you agree or disagree with the literature? Are your values within the ballpark?
- *Implications of your results.* In a separate paragraph.
- *Limitations of your study.* In a separate paragraph. Be honest!
- *Recommendations for future studies.* In a separate paragraph and should be the product of strong inference based on what you now know from your experiments. Strong inference here should be so obvious that someone should be able to guess the next experiment.

4.2.6.1   Additional hints for the discussion
Hint 1: Here is a nice discussion checklist adopted from Weiss (1995).

1. Did you discuss the results with respect to your hypotheses?
2. Did you discuss your findings with respect to those of previous studies in the literature?
3. Did you discuss the theoretical and practical implications of your findings?
4. Did you identify future directions for the work?
5. Did you state a clear take-home message?

Hint 2: You do not need to create a separate conclusions section (unless the journal requires it), but the final paragraph should leave the reader with your final message within the framework of the question, hypothesis, or purpose posed in the introduction. A Technical Note might end with a

[2] As a scientist, besides being meticulous, you have to be honest too. As I say to my students, if your middle name is meticulous, then your last name is honest!

statement regarding the novelty or utility of your approach. Ask yourself what you most want the reader to remember? Make sure this take-home message is clearly stated.

Hint 3: In his "Strong inference" article, Platt (1964) makes the following statement:

> The papers of the French leaders Francois Jacob and Jacques Monod are also celebrated for their high "logical density," with paragraph after paragraph of linked "inductive syllogisms." But the style is widespread. Start with the first paper in the Journal of Molecular Biology for 1964, and you immediately find: "Our conclusions... might be invalid if...(i)... (ii)...or (iii)...We shall describe experiments which eliminate these alternatives."
>
> *(Platt, 1964; page 348).*

It is powerful to point out the problems related to your study and, additionally, state solutions to those specific problems. Here is an example of how can you accomplish this, adopted from one of the papers that I published (Chien et al., 2017):

> Our experimental design, and the results produced, could guide a more sensitive screening of vestibular system deterioration. Before such clinical translational efforts are made, however, the above conclusions should be tested by replication of our experiments with: over ground walking during which visual, somatosensory, and vestibular manipulations are introduced without the restrictions of the treadmill; galvanic vestibular stimulation, dorsal neck muscles vibrations[39,40], or changing head posture, known to affect balance and orientation responses[41,42]. These experiments will allow us to eliminate alternative hypotheses pertaining to the effect of the apparatus and the differences that exist between mastoid vibration and other stimulations to vestibular inputs.
>
> *(Chien et al., 2017, www.nature.com/articles/srep41547)*

4.3   General tips on effective writing

The most important characteristic of effective scientific writing is a compelling story. This is achieved by the thrill of following out a chain of reasoning. It is similar to the thrill of following a detective story. The master of such writing is Sir Conan Doyle.

In the introduction, you spoke about the crime and you got your readers all excited with puzzles and suspense. You introduce your characters; your brilliant Sherlock Holmes, your sympathetic Inspector Lestrades, and the admiring Doctor Watson. In the methods, you place the inspector in the crime scene, examining every detail. Such details provide the reader with confidence about the ultimate resolution of the mystery. In the results, you have the climax: the important findings that the detective uncovered are presented. Finally, in the discussion, you provide a feeling of resolution, tying up all loose ends as you resolve whatever conflict was created by your results. The detective pulls all of the information together and the reader is enlightened. However, you also introduce the next "episode" as you present the next experiments in your logical tree (Ness, 2007).

This is why I recommend my students to take a writing class, even just a part-time one. The kind where you learn to convey vision, tension, conflict and solutions succinctly and rapidly can be especially useful. A beginners' screenwriting class could also be beneficial, short stories, poetry; whatever would help you learn to communicate your vision to others. As I said, creating your manuscript is a little like storytelling, so literature writing classes can actually really help with your scientific writing. Reading fiction can also be helpful for your writing skills. When I was a PhD student, my mentor forced us to read a huge amount of books and papers.

4.3.1   Additional general hints for effective writing

Hint 1: Brevity is a virtue. Say as much as you have to illustrate your logic and convince readers that your interpretation is correct – but not one word more. Rambling is the enemy of suspense.

Hint 2: Remember the basics. Paragraphs should begin with a topic sentence and contain only information on that topic. Write in an active voice; instead of writing, "It was found," go ahead and say who found it: "We found," or "They found." You can't tell a good crime story without detectives.

Hint 3: Writing well comes from writing a lot. Some writers begin with an outline, and others don't. Some write everything in their head, and others begin to formulate the story only after sitting down to type. *No matter what technique you use, good papers require dozens of drafts. So get comfortable with your computer.*

Hint 4: It is very easy to write a manuscript! Write an introduction by justifying the study. Put some people in front of you and explain your justification to them of why you are doing your study. Record yourself and all of a sudden you have a draft of your introduction.

4.4 The cover letter

I personally always include a cover letter because it gives you a chance to justify why your study is related to the mission and vision statement of the specific journal you are applying to (Vignettes 4.1 and 4.2). In addition, it gives you a chance to mention which reviewers you want to include and which ones you want to exclude. If you're the first to introduce a new variable or approach to the editors who have never published a paper in that specific area, you need to justify and explain everything in order to make it easy for them to understand. The cover letter gives you the opportunity to explain why, despite the unfamiliar-sounding material, approach or variables, you have chosen to target that specific journal (see especially Vignette 4.2 for an example). Nowadays, a lot of manuscripts that are submitted to good journals, do not even make it past the editor. If the editor deems your paper "out of purpose," it will not be sent to the reviewers and it will not be published. A detailed cover letter can help to overcome this first hurdle and move your manuscript to the reviewers.

VIGNETTE 4.1   Sample cover letter 1

"Dear Dr. …, *[the Editor in Chief of the journal]*

Please find enclosed an original scientific manuscript titled "…" that we would like to submit to your prestigious journal for review and publication consideration. This manuscript represents original material that is unpublished except in abstract form, and not under consideration for publication elsewhere. Further, it will not be submitted for publication elsewhere until a decision is made regarding its acceptability for publication in TITLE OF THE JOURNAL. If accepted for publication, I agree that it will not be published elsewhere, in whole or in part, without the consent of TITLE OF THE JOURNAL. In addition, there is no conflict of interest or endorsement of products by the authors. The typescripts have been read and agreed by all authors.

I and my co-authors have elected to submit this manuscript to TITLE OF THE JOURNAL because … (EXPLAIN HOW YOUR PAPER RELATES TO THE MISSION OF THE JOURNAL).

Furthermore, we would like to ask you to exclude XXXXXXXXX as a potential reviewer. Thank you in advance for your consideration. All correspondence should be directed to Dr. Nick Stergiou at the address provided below."

VIGNETTE 4.2   Sample cover letter 2

"Dear Dr. ..., *[the Editor in Chief of the journal]*

Please find enclosed an original research paper titled "..." that I and the other authors would like to submit to the Journal of ... for review and publication consideration. This manuscript represents original unpublished material, except in abstract form, that is not under consideration for publication elsewhere. Further, it will not be submitted for publication elsewhere until a decision is made regarding its acceptability for publication in the Journal of .... If accepted for publication, I agree that it will not be published elsewhere, in whole or in part, without the consent of the Journal of .... In addition, there is no conflict of interest or endorsement of products by the authors. The typescripts have been read and agreed by all authors. Furthermore, we would like to ask you to exclude Dr. XXXXXXXXX as a potential reviewer.

The work presented in this manuscript is the result of collaboration between physical therapists at the University of Nebraska Medical Center and biomechanists at the University of Nebraska at Omaha. We believe that using the information theory concept of "entropy" to describe randomness in sitting postural control in infants, we gain a unique perspective on the motor pathology of cerebral palsy. The interaction and synergy of our collaboration between the more mathematically focused biomechanists and the more clinically focused physical therapists is what makes this work unique. We have elected to submit this manuscript to the Journal of ... because we believe it fits well with the stated objectives of this journal; to promote cross-fertilization between the disciplines, and use concepts from other disciplines to help reshape physical medicine and rehabilitation. Thank you for your consideration of this work. All correspondence should be directed to Dr. Nick Stergiou, at the address provided below."

4.4.1   *Suggesting or excluding potential reviewers*

When authors suggest reviewers, the acceptance rate increases and the rejection rate decreases (Grimm, 2005). For example, a 9-month survey of 788 reviews for 329 manuscripts found no significant difference in the quality or timeliness of reviews between editor-suggested reviewers and author-suggested reviewers. However, they did find that *author-suggested reviewers were more likely to recommend manuscript publication* (55.7% versus 49.5%) *and less likely to recommend rejection* (14.4% versus 24.1%). In another study, author-suggested reviewers were more likely to advocate manuscript acceptance (47% versus 35%) and less likely to recommend rejection (10% versus 23%) (Grimm, 2005). There is a major difference in rejection rates between the two groups: ~10% difference between author- and editor-suggested reviewers. Opting to exclude reviewers may have an even more dramatic effect on a manuscript's success. In a study published in the *Journal of Investigative Dermatology*, for example, in 228 consecutive manuscript submissions in 2003, the authors found that the odds of acceptance were twice as high for manuscripts for which authors had excluded reviewers compared to those whose authors had not done so (Grimm, 2005). Just by excluding reviewers, the acceptance rate was doubled! This shows that as an author you have the power to increase your success rate (Grimm, 2005).

4.5 The references – citing the literature in your manuscript

At the end of your manuscript you include your references. Make sure that your list is comprehensive. Make sure you have read extensively to develop a thorough knowledge (so you can also develop your logical tree). I have recently seen several authors publish manuscripts with findings that we've known since the 1980s. This is especially true in the running biomechanics that I am quite familiar with. Make a habit of reading all the journals pertinent to your field at least once a month. Scan the titles and then get the important ones for your work. Set up searches in PubMed or other search engines with your keywords.

It is also important to be aware of what are called *primary* and *secondary* references. Primary references provide the original findings and are reported by the people who did the study or experiment. Secondary references involve somebody else's description of those findings. Relying on secondary references creates problems. If the secondary author portrays the results inaccurately or omits crucial details, associated findings, interpretations or study limitations, your Strong Inference and logical tree may be affected. These secondary results have been subjected to another person's bias and opinion, and interpretations may be different when they transfer from one person to another. If journal reviewers spot secondary references, your papers will be denied. And quite rightly. I have seen this case multiple times. The solution is to get the primary references and read them for yourself.

4.6 What is the impact of your published manuscript?

In general, you increase the impact of your research if you publish in journals that have a higher impact factor. The impact factor of a journal is a measure reflecting the yearly average number of citations to recent articles published in that journal. There are a number of publications regarding the value of the impact factor (Hoeffel, 1998; Garfield, 2006). However, there are also a number of publications that heavily criticize the impact factor (Callaway, 2016; van Wesel, 2016; Brembs et al., 2013). Some take these numbers very seriously (e.g. funding agencies). It's visibility. My advice is to try to publish your work in journals that have higher impact factor if you are able to (see Table 4.1 for some examples). On the other hand, if you don't publish at all, then *your study never happened*. Your work doesn't exist. Your priority should be to publish your work, even in a lower impact journal. Never forget that the seminal publication of Edward Lorenz in 1963 that introduced Chaos theory. It did not immediately attract attention beyond his own field as it was published in the *Journal of the Atmospheric Sciences*, which was a fairly low impact journal and not widely read. However, by the mid-1970s, with the rise of similar work by Bernard Mandelbrot and others, the "butterfly effect" that was introduced by Lorenz, had become a subject of debate. It seemed to affect a wide range of academic disciplines, and Lorenz's paper began to be cited regularly (Lorenz, 1963). *Research that is not published in any form has no impact.*

Another issue to consider is whether the journal that you plan to submit to, and eventually have your manuscript published in, appears in search engines. In the present day, we rely heavily on search engines to find pertinent literature. This is because of the large volume of publications that are produced. If the journal you publish in is not listed by these search engines, your article cannot be found. It is therefore essential to publish in journals that are listed by search engines that are relevant to your field. For example, my number one search engine is PubMed. PubMed includes more than 29 million citations for biomedical literature from MEDLINE, life science journals, and online books (www.ncbi.nlm. nih.gov/pubmed/). I need to publish my paper in journals that are listed by PubMed. Otherwise it may be missed entirely by people in my field.

Table 4.1 Impact Factors from a Range of Scientific Journals

Publication	Two-year impact factor
New England Journal of Medicine	72.406
Nature	40.137
Science	37.205
Cell	30.410
Nature Scientific Reports	4.259
Journal of Biomechanics	2.664
Experimental Brain Research	1.917

Journal metrics for 2016

Furthermore, submitting to an appropriate journal will allow you to disseminate your results faster. Choose a journal that has a mission that is a good fit for your work. If you have included multiple references from a specific journal, then it makes sense to submit your manuscript there.[3]

4.7   Additional publishing tips

4.7.1 When do I publish?

As you progress with your data collections, you need to decide when you have enough there to start crafting your manuscript. If you wait too long there is every chance that someone will get there first! Of course, this does not necessarily mean that other people are stealing your idea (See Vignette 4.3). If you've thought of something, it's very likely that someone else in this world will have thought of it too. *Remember that you are not the only smart person in this planet. There are a lot of smart people in the world. Hence, you may not be able to outsmart everyone, but you can outwork everybody.*

VIGNETTE 4.3   Avoiding predators

You *do* have to be careful about predators, because people *can* steal your ideas. You have to be careful of what you present during meetings and conferences. Someone may see your idea on your poster and publish it before you do. Make sure that the research work you present, is already protected by a published paper. At least, if you did not publish the paper, try to publish it as soon as possible. You have to be careful of what you mention in your website and newsletters. If we present our ideas to a company, they have to sign a nondisclosure agreement in order to prevent any leaking of information. You may want to consider doing the same, at least at a smaller scale. I tell my students that ethics comes from the heart, so if someone comes and presents a novel idea to you and you choose to make it your own then it is unethical. On the other hand, if you really like the idea then you should speak with this scientist and you can try to explore if you can collaborate and create something new. In general, I find scientists very open to collaborations especially in our times.

---

[3] I actually don't write for specific journals – I write to write. I first write the paper, and then find a journal that fits my paper's criteria. Choice of journal should also depend on your references. For example, if you have ten papers from the *Journal of Theoretical Biology* mentioned in your references, then you should probably publish it there.

4.7.2   *How do you know if it is too soon?*

Statistics will help direct your research with calculations of sample size and statistical power. For example, if your sample size justification calls for 40 subjects to collect because you did not have strong preliminary data to base your sample size estimations, you first collect 10 subjects and recalculate your sample size. You may realize that now your sample size is sufficient and you have sufficient power. If your data require complex processing before your statistical analysis, don't wait until the last minute to process all the data. You may have several errors. Take "time outs" from collecting data in order to process or try to process the data while collecting simultaneously. Furthermore, consider if your data tell a complete story. What figures can you already create? What information do they portray? Do they lead the reader to the same conclusion that you have arrived at? Remember your logical tree. Is there an alternative explanation for your results? Do you need to perform further experiments to eliminate it? Keep in mind that *there are no studies with no limitations*. These should be mentioned in the last section of your paper as we already mentioned above.

You can also seek advice from your colleagues. As you have been living and breathing your project every day, it is often difficult to be able to identify any inconsistencies or gaps in your logic. Try presenting your figures to a colleague and explaining your thought process surrounding them, and ask for honest feedback on whether they were convinced or not.

You also want to submit a high-quality paper. Poor quality writing implies poor quality science. Even if you designed and performed your experiment perfectly, if your writing is careless it will undermine all of the hard work you put in previously. This means that the logic must be crystal clear, the figures must be extremely neat and beautiful (axes labeled correctly and explicitly), and the writing majestic with no orthographical errors. Careless writing will reflect badly on you, your mentor or student, and the laboratory.

4.7.3   *Surviving the review process*

So you've got your review back from the journal. What do you do? Make sure you help the review process by providing a cover letter that details concisely the content of the paper and portrays its importance. Then, respond appropriately to reviewers' comments. Assume that the reviewers are offering constructive criticism rather than trying to attack you. Try your best to comply with their requests; or at least meet them half-way (see also chapter three). Be respectful. Never argue with them, and try not to use any negative terms (e.g. *disagree, disapprove,* etc.). I recently started publishing a lot with a friend of mine. Before submission, he sends me his *Responses to reviewers' comments* texts. They are always full of negative language. I end up fixing all the argumentative verbs and replace them with gentler language.

4.7.4   How do you deal with rejection?

Don't do something you might regret! The worst thing you can do after receiving a rejection is to send an incensed email off to the editor. Wait a day, take a time out, and reevaluate. After you've calmed down, if you feel that there has been an error or a misunderstanding somewhere along the process, express this. Occasionally your article may be reconsidered by the journal if you write a respectful letter explaining where you believe this has occurred.

Here is an interesting story. Previously, I received a major grant from the National Institute of Disability and Rehabilitation Research. The very first aim of that grant was to assess the reliability of nonlinear analysis techniques for both typically developing children and for children at risk of developmental disorders. We collected a lot of data during multiple sessions. After finishing the sessions with typically developing children, we wrote a paper and sent it to Archives of Physical Medicine and Rehabilitation. They rejected the manuscript even though the experiments and analyses were performed correctly. Even the comments were easily addressable. So, I wrote a very nice letter and sent it to the Editor in Chief explaining this. In addition, I suggested that it would be beneficial if they accepted manuscripts that were funded through grants from their own premiere funding agency. The rejection was lifted and a resubmission was allowed. We resubmitted and the manuscript was eventually published. This has actually happened to me several times during my career.

I have had countless rejections in my career, but I also have published more than 200 peer-reviewed scientific manuscripts. Thus, imagine how many rejections I have experienced in my career! Being frequently rejected in academia and science is a very demeaning experience, although it is very humbling as well. You will be rejected a lot, especially if you are presenting a new idea, a new method, or a new theoretical model. Benoit Mandelbrot was initially ridiculed for his pioneer work on fractals by other mathematicians and was called a "tinker-toy scientist." Now he is considered a scientific giant!

4.7.5   Teaching improves research writing in graduate students

Science, technology, engineering, and mathematics (STEM) graduate students are often encouraged to maximize their engagement with supervised research and to minimize teaching obligations. However, the process of teaching students also provides practice in the application of important research skills. A 2011 study published in *Science* (Feldon et al., 2011) compared the quality of methodological skills demonstrated in written research proposals for two groups of early career graduate students; those with both teaching and research responsibilities, and those with only research responsibilities, at the beginning and end of an academic year. After statistically controlling for preexisting differences between groups, students who both taught and conducted research demonstrated a significantly greater improvement in their abilities to generate testable hypotheses and design valid experiments.

When you teach, you have to learn how to explain complex material. This will lead to better development of your ideas. Most importantly, the courses you teach need to correspond to your research interest. You will not benefit in this way from teaching a yoga or a Classics course if your research interest relates to assessing asymmetrical movement in a post total knee arthroplasty population. On the other hand, teaching undergraduate biomechanics will help improve your skills and knowledge, especially if you talk about your research papers in class. Do not stay away from teaching because you think that it will consume your time and steer you away from research; rather seek opportunities to teach (as long as you do not have to teach an excessive amount of courses). Moreover, teaching will help improve your confidence and presentation skills.

4.7.6   *Choosing the right environment for writing*

When exploring the next step in their careers, most graduate students/ young faculty will examine the facilities that an institution houses. Others may visit sites in major cities just because it may be nice to live in them (e.g. Manhattan, Los Angeles, and Miami). Before deciding which environment to join, also *make sure to ask about the writing process*. As a graduate student (PhD or Masters), one of the most important decisions to make involves choosing an environment that will be good for publishing. The best way for you to learn to write first-class papers is by getting as much practice as possible. The more practice you have, the better you become.

Thus, in the environment you choose to attend for your graduate education or your postdoc experience, are you going to write the first draft of the manuscripts for publication? As a graduate student, your first draft will have plenty of mistakes, which is perfectly normal. The practice you get at making these mistakes and correcting them is essential in improving your writing skills. If your mentor always writes the first draft, then you will not have any chance to practice.

Do you get valuable feedback and guidance on their manuscripts? When? Many mentors provide input several months after they receive the draft, and sometimes the input is not valuable. For that reason, you have to be absolutely sure that the environment you want to join has mentors that are able to provide the time and the effort to help you improve your writing skills.

Are the papers that the mentor/laboratory produces in journals you would want to publish in? If you feel compelled to publish in the *Journal of Biomechanics* and the mentor in the desired environment only publishes in the *Journal of Experimental Psychology*, then you may be in the wrong place.

Also, you don't want to join a team that has the head of the laboratory as the first author in all of the published papers, or that appears to favor a specific individual (although, that individual could be working more than others; in that case we would need to investigate the case). Make sure to check that different members of the laboratory are listed as first author.

Search for the papers published by the mentor you want to study under. Don't just examine the publication record during your potential mentor's PhD education, but rather look at the publication record when he/she started working alone. It is possible that your potential mentor had excellent amount of training and many publications during the PhD or postdoc years because he/she was working under a demanding mentor, but that's only due to the external motivation provided by the mentor. You will not be publishing a lot if you move to an environment in which the mentor publishes one paper a year. You have to be absolutely sure that you will have both the time and the opportunity to publish papers in the environment that you choose to relocate to.

4.7.7   Writing help

I have included below some specific help in terms of writing.

For continuing a common line of reasoning: consequently, furthermore, additionally, also, and, in addition to, moreover, because, besides that, in the same way, again, couples with, similarly, likewise

To change line of reasoning: however, on the other hand, but, yet, nevertheless, on the contrary, despite

Contrast and comparison: conversely, instead, likewise, on one hand, on the other hand, on the contrary, rather, similarly, yet, but, however, still, nevertheless, in contrast

Emphasis: above all, chiefly, with attention to, especially, particularly, singularly

Exemplifying: chiefly, especially, for instance, in particular, markedly, namely, particularly, including, specifically, such as

Exception: aside from, barring, beside, except, excepting, excluding, exclusive of, other than, outside of, save

Consequence: accordingly, as a result, consequently, for this reason, for this purpose, hence, otherwise, so then, subsequently, therefore, thus, thereupon

Generalizing: as a rule, as usual, for the most part, generally, generally speaking, ordinarily, usually

Illustration: for example, for instance, for one thing, as an illustration, illustrated with, as an example, in this case

Similarity: comparatively, coupled with, correspondingly, identically, likewise, similar, moreover, together with

Restatement: in essence, in other words, namely, that is, that is to say, in short, in brief

Sequence: at first, first of all, to begin with, in the first place, at the same time, for now, for the time being, the next step, in time, in turn, later on, meanwhile, next, then, soon, the meantime, later, while, earlier, simultaneously, afterward, in conclusion, with this in mind

Transition chains/chronological arrangement

- First … Second … Third
- Generally … Furthermore … Finally
- In the first place … Also … Lastly
- In the first place … Pursuing this further … Finally
- To be sure … Additionally … Lastly
- In the first place … Just in the same way … Finally
- Basically … Similarly … As well

The above are from the following three books; these books are extremely valuable in terms of writing:

Casagrande, J. (2010). *It Was the Best of Sentences, It Was the Worst of Sentences*. The Ten Speed Press.

Glasman-Deal, H. (2010). *Science Research Writing*. Imperial College Press.

Greene, A.E. (2013). *Writing Science in Plain English*. The University of Chicago Press.

References

Brembs, B., Button, K., Munafò, M. (2013). Deep impact: unintended consequences of journal rank. *Frontiers in Human Neuroscience*, 7(291), 1–12.

Callaway, E. (2016). Beat it, impact factor! Publishing elite turns against controversial metric. *Nature*, 535(7611), 210–211.

Chien, J.H., Mukherjee, M., Kent, J., Stergiou, N. (2017). Mastoid vibration affects dynamic postural control during gait in healthy older adults. *Nature Scientific Reports*, 7, 41547.

Feldon, D.F., Peugh, J., Timmerman, B.E., Maher, M.A., Hurst, M., Strickland, D., Gilmore, J.A., Stiegelmeyer, C. (2011). Graduate students' teaching experiences improve their methodological research skills. *Science*, 333(6045), 1037–1039.

Garfield, E. (2006). The history and meaning of the journal impact factor. *JAMA,* 295(1), 90–93.

Grimm, D. (2005). Peer review. Suggesting or excluding reviewers can help get your paper published. *Science,* 309(5743), 1974.

Hoeffel, C. (1998). Journal impact factors. *Allergy,* 53(12), 1225.

Ness, R. (2007). Writing science: the story's the thing. *Science.* doi:10.1126/science.caredit.a0700047.

Platt, J.R. (1964). Strong inference. Certain systematic methods of scientific thinking may produce much more rapid progress than others. *Science,* 146(3642), 347–353.

van Wesel, M. (2016). Evaluation by citation: trends in publication behavior, evaluation criteria, and the strive for high impact publications. *Science and Engineering Ethics,* 22(1), 199–225.

Weiss, M.R. (1995). Editor's viewpoint: Do you know the way to San Jose. *Research Quarterly for Exercise and Sport,* 66(1), iii–v.

Additional Readings

Kelner, K. (2007). Tips for publishing in scientific journals. *Science.* doi:10.1126/science.caredit.a0700046.

Lorenz, E. N. (1963). Deterministic Nonperiodic Flow. *Journal of Atmospheric Sciences,* 20, 130–141.

Nancekivell, N. (2004). Writing a publishable journal article: a perspective from the other side of the desk. *Science.* Retrieved from www.sciencemag.org/careers/2004/04/writing-publishable-journal-article-perspective-other-side-desk.

Sternberg, R. J. (2008). How to win acceptances by psychology journals: 21 tips for better writing. *Pan-Pacific Management Review,* 11(1), 51–59.

Weiss, M.R. (1994). Editor's viewpoint: why ask "why?". *Research Quarterly for Exercise and Sport,* 65(1), iii–v.

Wright, T.M., Buckwalter, J.A., Hayes, W.C. (1999). Writing for the journal of orthopedic research. *Journal of Orthopedic Research,* 17(4), 459–466.

chapter five

Ethics

> It is the mark of an educated mind to be able to entertain a thought without accepting it.
>
> **—Aristotle (384–322 BC)**

5.1   Introduction

This chapter provides information about responsible conduct of research. Several topics are presented including those related to authorship, supervisory and mentoring relationships, and other scientific tasks.

5.2   Responsible conduct in research

So why does responsible conduct in research really matter? There are several reasons, but I believe the most important one is that there is no room for misconduct in the search for "truth." In addition, it reinforces public support of science, protects research subjects, maintains integrity of the scientific process, and it is just the right thing to do. But what is research misconduct? Research misconduct is defined as fabrication, falsification, or plagiarism in proposing, performing, or reviewing research, or in reporting research results (Office of Science and Technology Policy, 2000). Fabrication means making up data or results and recording or reporting them. Falsification refers to manipulating research materials, equipment, or processes, or changing or omitting data or results such that the research is not accurately represented in the research record. Plagiarism is the appropriation of another person's research ideas, processes, results, or words without giving appropriate credit. Research misconduct does not include honest error or differences of opinion (Office of Science and Technology Policy, 2000). Honest error is an error that occurs due to the malfunction of an instrument or the inappropriate use of a technique, whereas misconduct error occurs intentionally, knowingly, and recklessly.

You would be wise to familiarize yourself with the Office of Research Integrity that oversees and directs Public Health Service research integrity activities on behalf of the Secretary of Health and Human Services. An exception to their oversight are the regulatory research integrity activities of the Food and Drug Administration. On their website (https://ori.hhs.gov/), you can find the most recent cases of research misconduct, along with many summaries of cases that have occurred in previous years (https://ori.hhs.gov/case_summary). In general, cases of research misconduct involve all disciplines, even Nobel Prize winners. Nobody is immune, and this is why it is very important to be extremely careful. Here are some examples of research misconduct that have made headlines over the years:

- Marc Hauser was a Harvard University professor from 1998 to 2011, when he resigned after being found guilty for research misconduct. His studies included work on the cognitive and evolutionary underpinning of language. Former graduate students raised allegations which resulted in a 3-year investigation that found Hauser had fabricated data, manipulated experimental results, and published falsified findings. His famous 2002 paper in the journal Cognition was retracted. In this paper, Hauser and his collaborators concluded that cotton-top tamarin monkeys could learn simple rule-like patterns (Wade, 2010).
- Linda Buck is an American biologist, best known for her work on the olfactory system. She was awarded the 2004 Nobel Prize in Physiology. In 2008, she retracted a 2001 *Nature* paper after noticing inconsistencies between some of the figures and data published in the paper and the original data. Buck also retracted two more papers (one published in *Proceedings of the National Academy of Sciences* (*PNAS*) in 2005 and the other in *Science* in 2006). The Office of Research Integrity found that Zhihua Zou, a postdoc in Buck's lab at Harvard Medical School who was the lead author on all three papers, was guilty of research misconduct. The investigation showed that Zou falsified several figures in the *Nature* paper and one figure in the *PNAS* paper. The retracted material was not related to Buck's 2004 Nobel Prize (Chang, 2010).
- Scott S. Reuben was a professor of Anesthesiology at Tufts University in Boston from February, 1991, until 2009. He is currently in prison for healthcare fraud. He was considered as one of the most prolific researchers in anesthesiology and pain management. In what is called the "longest-running and widest ranging case of academic fraud ever," Reuben admitted that he never conducted any of the clinical trials that resulted in 21 journal articles since 1999 and the efficacy of use of neuropathic pain medicines instead of narcotics is now widely questioned. An anonymous colleague said about Reuben: "Interestingly, when you look at Scott's output over the last 15 years, he never had a negative study. In fact, they were all

very robust results – where others had failed to show much difference. I don't understand how anyone could pull this off for so long!"
(Harris, 2009).

Here are two additional examples of research misconduct in the movement sciences involving highly respected scientists:

- Thomas Pipes was a student under the direction of legendary
  exercise physiologist Jack Wilmore. He completed a study that was
  published in *Medicine and Science in Sports and Exercise*. The results
  were challenged by Richard Berger. Wilmore decided to send the
  data to Berger for reanalysis. Therefore, he asked his student to get
  him the actual raw data. However, the student refused, and a month
  later, Wilmore submitted a statement of withdrawal to the journal
  and a retraction was published (Wilmore, 1979).
- Fred Daniels was a doctoral student of Dan Landers at Arizona
  State University. Some of the other students noticed that he was
  completing his work extremely fast and they started to question
  his data. More allegations were made regarding his score sheets,
  and, eventually, Daniels admitted to Landers and his colleagues
  that he had fabricated the data. Daniels was dismissed from the
  university. Furthermore, it was found that Daniels followed similar practices while performing his master's thesis at Penn State
  University under Bob Christina. This led to the withdrawal
  of Daniels's thesis, the removal of all A grades for his research
  courses, and the publication of retractions (Landers and Christina,
  1986; Daniels 1985).

Wilmore, Christina, and Daniels were highly respected movement
scientists; but as I mentioned earlier, nobody is immune. What we need
to do is to make every possible effort to ensure that ethical practices are
followed in our research. It helps to retain a sense of humility, knowing
that we can also be deceived.

5.3 Authorship

Starting from the early 1960s, we have had an explosion of scientific
literature. A quick search on Medline shows that we went from 200,000
scientific papers in 1970 to 500,000 in 2000. This is compounded by the
proliferation of authors per paper. For example, in Lancet we went from
two authors per paper in 1950 to five authors per paper in 2000. These
numbers are increasing rapidly. An extreme example of authorship is a
paper on the genome sequence of drosophila melanogaster published in

Science at 2000. There were 195 authors overall! The first author, Adams, was followed by 30 other authors in an unknown relational order. This was followed by 159 other authors in alphabetical order: from Abril to Zhu. This was followed by five "senior authors" which were Smith, Gibbs, Myers, Rubin, and Venter (the "most senior" of the "seniors"). Interestingly 34 organizations were listed.

The above trends have increased the number of issues of research misconduct in authorship. The most common of them are (a) Duplicate Papers, (b) Authorship Disputes, (c) Authorship Proliferation, (d) Honorary Authorship, (e) Specific Roles of Authors, and (f) Falsification, Fabrication, and Plagiarism. I will present some of these issues below.

5.3.1 Why do we have problems with authorship?

Here is a short list of some reasons.

More scientists and clinical researchers ask for your skills. For example, there are clinicians and other scientists who ask for my evaluation of biomechanical data or want to add biomechanical data into their study and so on.

There is a need to collaborate. Technology is becoming more and more complex, and multidisciplinary projects frequently require specialist knowledge from a range of different fields. Researchers, for example, may want to apply the non-linear analysis techniques in which I specialize. It is also mandatory to have a team when you submit a grant. This means that there will be more people working on a project.

Less tenure-track positions and more applicants. Over 300 applicants may apply for a tenure track position when it is offered in psychology. Similar cases are seen in mathematics and chemistry. On the other hand, even though we don't face these issues in biomechanics, we still compete with biomedical engineers, kinesiologists, and biologists for positions. To be able to get a faculty position and attain tenure, you need to build an impressive résumé, and publications are a huge part of this.

Funding budgets do not change, but more people are applying for funding. The National Institutes of Health (NIH) budget does not increase based on how many people apply. If we correlate the budget of the NIH with the number of applications delivered per year, there will not be a 1:1 correlation. The budget trajectory is normally flat in comparison with the grant applications received. Therefore, competition is fierce, and, again, a better résumé may help you to get funding.

There is a businesslike approach to academia regarding receiving R01 funding and securing indirect cost. Nowadays, we witness a business-like approach in academia. Many funding sources require a *biosketch*;

a succinct standard-form CV that displays your work output alongside how you have contributed to science. Scientists are obligated to publish more papers in order to compile and flaunt impressive biosketches. If you do not have a good biosketch, you cannot attain external funding. Funding brings in indirect costs to the university. If we include the salaries that are funded by large grants, the university gains a whole lot more. Usually, full-time faculty members are hired to obtain external funding and not to teach. They are paid, as an example, $80,000 per year, while part-time faculty members are only paid $5,000 per course. Thus, the university thinks that it is more economical to hire part-time professors to teach. In comparison, the full-time professors teach very little (one class per semester), and their job is mostly focused on obtaining external funding. This funding provides the university the full-time professors' salaries plus the salaries of the part-time teachers through the acquired indirect costs. This is a very good financial model for the universities, but it means that the full-time professors really need to obtain external funding to improve their chances to get accolades (i.e. tenure and promotion). It is unsurprising that full-time professors want their names to be included on as many papers as possible; a good biosketch will give them a better chance of receiving this funding.

5.3.2 Determining authorship credit

This is a very important issue that continuously creates friction in academia. You will face it if you haven't faced it already. At the end of last century, for example, the Ombuds Office of Harvard Medical School and its associated hospitals reported an increase in disputes such that over 10% of the issues that were brought to them were over authorship (Wilcox, 1998); that is, someone was not included on an authorship that should have been, or someone received undeserved credit. Note, these were the *recorded* issues. They had no knowledge of those that were not recorded. The topic of authorship is unavoidable and will continually be problematic if *ego* keeps consuming our lives. Therefore, it is important to agree on authorship rules and order of the authors on the publication, before you start conducting the study. This will ease the process, and everyone will be certain of their roles and contributions. However, a critical question is: Who should receive authorship? Who do you think should be an author on a scientific paper? Let us list some cases that could cause problems:

- *I'm the lab director – What about me?* Many lab directors feel the need to be mentioned as an author just because of their title. I am aware of large laboratories around the world where more than 100 people work on a variety of topics within the same environment. In several of these places, their lab directors demand that their name is on every publication. They may be completely unfamiliar with the experiments that the different research teams perform but still want to receive authorship.

- *I'm in the lab group – What about me?* Graduate students who are involved in a research team, for example, may think they can gain authorship, even if they did not contribute to the research study.
- *I'm the department chair – What about me?* Again, people may feel the need to be mentioned in a paper just because of their title.
- *You used my technology – What about me?* Someone may have built a piece of equipment that is used within a study, for example, and feel the need to be mentioned as an author in the paper just because of that.
- *I critiqued the paper – What about me?* Because of providing feedback while reviewing the manuscript, a person may feel that they should be mentioned as an author.
- *I'm your best friend – What about me?!!*
- *I'm your wife – What about me?!!*

5.3.3   Who should get authorship?

For years, I have been posing this question to my graduate students, postdocs, and young faculty. The following are what they consider as important:

- *The person who has the idea?*
- *The person who collected the data?*
- *The person who processed the data?*
- *The person who analyzed the data?*
- *The person who wrote the paper?*
- *The person who revised the paper?*

We should mention that faculty members tend to weigh more on the idea and the writing, while graduate students on data collection, processing, and analysis. Of course, this doesn't surprise anyone. So, let us explore this question, on who should get authorship, more closely. Four excellent hypothetical cases are presented here, adopted from the publication of Fine and Kurdek (1993). We relist them and provide the results of an in-class discussion with my students, along with the authors' proposed solution.

VIGNETTE 5.1 Case 1

"A clinical psychology student conducted her PhD dissertation research at the site where she had completed her practicum. The student's dissertation committee consisted of two faculty members in the student's graduate department, one of whom was chair, plus the practicum supervisor. The practicum supervisor and the student developed the initial idea for the study. It was suggested by the chair that a journal article be written based on the student's dissertation work, for which the student agreed to write all drafts, with the chair supervising and the practicum supervisor reviewing. The student would be granted first author, and the practicum and committee chair second and third authors, respectively. The student later acknowledged that she had lost interest and the committee chair completed and submitted the work, after performing an extensive reanalysis of the data."

The authors' solution: The student deserved to be listed on the authorship given her contributions, which included the development of the research design, writing the research proposal, data collection and manuscript drafting. Her position in the authorship list is less straightforward, as the manuscript was completed by the faculty member due to the student's loss of interest. Listing the student in first author position despite this would be dependent on whether the collaborators had previously agreed that this would happen, even if she didn't fulfill her responsibilities. Similarly, the credit given to the practicum supervisor should depend on the extent to which he fulfilled the professional responsibilities he had previously agreed upon with respect to the article.

What do my students think? It was unanimously agreed that the student, the committee chair, and the practicum supervisor needed to be included as authors in the final paper as they had all made important contributions. As for the order, the students had different ideas and opinions. Some felt that the student should retain first author position as it was a manuscript based on her dissertation. A few stated that the practicum supervisor should be first, followed by the student, with the committee chair at anchor position, which might better reflect the committee chairs advisory role. Others disagreed and felt that the practicum supervisor should not be the first author, since he did not contribute enough to the study to warrant this honor. Several students agreed that the committee chair should be the first author since he performed a reanalysis and revised the work substantially prior to submission, after the student had lost interest.

VIGNETTE 5.2   Case 2

"A faculty member was asked to supervise the honors thesis of an undergraduate psychology student. After the student had proposed a topic for the thesis, the research methodology was primarily developed by the faculty member. Data was collected by the student. The statistical analyses were performed by the faculty member. A part of this analysis was used in the student's thesis, which was written under the supervision of the faculty member. The faculty member then decided that the project could be written up as a journal article. The faculty member wrote the journal article as the student did not have the necessary skills to do this. About a third of the content of the article was in the student's thesis."

The authors' solution: The student deserved authorship credit to some extent, as she provided the topic, helped to formulate the study design, and wrote her honors thesis. First authorship is another matter. If she had the desire and commitment to expand on the work of her thesis and take on the responsibilities of the task of writing the manuscript, then ethically the supervisor had the obligation to assist her in this. In this situation, she would have been given first authorship. If not, second authorship would be ethically appropriate, with first authorship granted to the supervisor. A footnote that indicated that part of the article was based on the honors thesis of the student might additionally be included.

What do my students think? There was a general consensus that, although the faculty member wrote the article, the student should have had first authorship because a large proportion was taken from his thesis. A few students expressed that they felt the student should have been given the opportunity to attempt writing a draft of the manuscript under supervision of the faculty member.

VIGNETTE 5.3   Case 3

"A psychologist and psychiatrist developed the design for a study. A student was later brought on to assist in the study, a portion of which would be his master's thesis. The student found additional pertinent literature and collected a proportion of the data and analyzed it. The thesis was written under the supervision of the psychologist. After completion of the

> thesis, the psychologist and psychiatrist wrote up certain sections of the study into a journal article, following additional analysis. The student was not asked to contribute."

The authors' solution: Although the contributions of the student were minimal, they would be considered professional, at least cumulatively, warranting third authorship. He gathered additional literature upon the titles already identified, collected data, performed some analysis, and wrote his master's thesis. He did not contribute in terms of the research idea and design, or in the manuscript-writing process, and was therefore lacking in these areas. In addition, further analyses were conducted by the supervisor.

What do my students think? Some argued that the student should have been included as an author; however, the majority agreed that the psychologist and psychiatrist should be the first and second authors, respectively, and it was right for the student not to be included. The failure to give the student the opportunity to contribute to the manuscript was again questioned, however.

VIGNETTE 5.4   Case 4

"The student chose the topic of her own undergraduate honors thesis. In a search, she determined that there were no suitable measures for the independent variables she wished to explore. Based on this, a new measure was developed jointly by the student and the faculty member supervising her project. Data collection and entry was performed by the student. The faculty member analyzed the data. The thesis was written by the student under the guidance of the faculty member, and it required few revisions. The faculty member wrote the journal article for the work, because the student did not have the skills to do so. The student was listed as first author. The first submission was returned by the reviewers requiring a major revision, which sought the addition of aspects of the study that were extraneous to the thesis."

The authors' solution: The student generated the topic herself and contributed in the study design and the development of the measurement technique, with little supervision. She clearly deserved authorship. She should have been given the opportunity to assist in revising the manuscript following review and, if she did so, would be deserving of first authorship.

What do my students think? Most agreed that both the student and the faculty member should be included as authors in the article and that the student should be given first author position.

5.3.4   What would the authorities say?

The American Psychological Association Ethics Committee states that dissertation supervisors should be included as authors on such articles only when they made "substantial contributions" to the study. The student should have first authorship. It is ethically poor for a faculty member to take an undeserved level of authorship credit and deny it to the student. It is equally unethical for students to be granted credit that they did not deserve, however. Such credit would be a misrepresentation of the individual's expertise, knowledge in a topic, or academic ability. This could potentially lead to an unfair advantage over unpublished peers or unrealistic expectations of their ability by future employers (APA, 1983).

Many journals publish, within their guidelines for authors, their requirements for authorship. For example, *Journal of the American Medical Association* (JAMA) lists the following requirements:

> All persons designated as authors should qualify for authorship. Each author should have participated sufficiently in the work to take public responsibility for the content.
>
> Authorship credit should be based only on substantial contributions to (1) conception and design or analysis and interpretation of the data; and to (2) drafting the article or revising it critically for important intellectual content; and to (3) final approval of the version to be published. Conditions 1, 2, and 3 must ALL be met. Participation solely in the acquisition of funding or the collection of data does not justify authorship. General supervision of the research group is not sufficient for authorship.
>
> The order of authorship should be a joint decision of the co-authors. Authors may wish to explain the order of authorship in a footnote.
>
> —*(JAMA 277:927, 1997)*

Some journals may require completion of a form similar to the one we see in Vignette 5.5 (http://jamanetwork.com/DocumentLibrary/InstructionsForAuthors/JAMA/auinst_crit.pdf):

VIGNETTE 5.5   Authorship form

I have made substantial contributions to the intellectual content of the paper as described below.

1. Check at least one of two below
   - Conception or design
   - Acquisition, analysis, or interpretation of data
2. Check at least one of two below
   - Drafting of the manuscript
   - Critical revision of the manuscript for important intellectual content
3. Check at least one below
   - Statistical analysis
   - Obtaining funding
   - Administrative, technical, or material support
   - Supervision
   - No additional contributions
   - Other

You need to have contributed with at least one item from each section to receive authorship. JAMA will send an email to each author in the study asking for their approval of the final manuscript to be published.

The Guidelines for the conduct of research in the Intramural Research Program at the NIH state:

> … individuals who have assisted in the research by their encouragement and advice or by providing space, financial support, reagents, occasional analyses or patient material should be acknowledged in the text, but not be authors

(EMBO Reports 5:446, 2004).

For example, one of your colleagues who continuously encourages you to strive for success (a nice thing to do), should not be an author (and probably not in the acknowledgements either). It's the same for your significant other! If someone reanalyzes a data set that was collected by another scientist and writes a paper based on that analysis, the authorship should depend on the prior agreement that was put in place.

5.3.5   Additional issues

5.3.5.1   Honorary authorship in major journals

Even though we have all the above guidelines, issues persist, and honorary authorship is common in the medical field. *Honorary* authorship is when an author is added for reasons other than their making a true contribution to the research. For example, an author may be added as a "thank you," or due to a professional (or personal) relationship with one or more of the authors. Table 5.1 shows the percentage of honorary authors in three general medical journals, and the percentage of articles with honorary authors, that is, those who would not meet the requirements of the International Committee of Medical Journal Editors (Bates et al., 2004). As you see, it could be a significant problem. It is even more of an issue in medical journals, where it is not unusual to see 20 or more names on the authorship of a manuscript.

5.3.5.2   Misrepresentation of authorship among applicants to training programs

If someone applies for a medical school, or upon completion of medical school, applies for a fellowship to gain further knowledge, a publication record may boost their application. Table 5.2 shows the numbers of applicants to medical schools in four disciplines that had invalid publications cited in their applications (selected years from 1992 to 1999). In the year 1995, for example, it was identified that from 404 applicants to pediatrics training programs, 19.7% of the publications listed were invalid. This is a major failure.

5.3.6   Managing authorship

Below is some advice for dealing with authorship and avoiding disputes.

- *Establish who's who early on in your research group.* Before starting a project in a research group, it is good practice to establish everyone's contributions. You should have that conversation to avoid any dispute from arising. While you are having this conversation, remember that being the "First Author" is still most important, being in the first few

Table 5.1 Honorary Authorships in Three General Medical Journals

	Authors (%)	Articles (%)
Annals of Internal Medicine	21.5	60
British Medical Journal (BMJ)	9.5	21
Journal of the American Medical Association (JAMA)	0.5	4

Source: Bates et al. (2004).
We assume that "final review and approval" is true for all three.

Table 5.2 Applicants to Training Programs Citing Invalid Publications

Reference	Discipline	Year(s)	No. of applicants	No. of applicants with publications	No. of publications in total	Publications invalid (%)
Acad Med 73:532, 1998	Pediatrics	1995	404	147	401	19.7
Am J Radiol 170:577, 1998	Radiology	1992–1995	201	87	261	15.0
Ann Int Med 123:38, 1995	Gastroenterology	1995	236	53	92	30.2
J Bone & Joint Surg 81A:1679, 1999	Orthopaedics	1998–1999	213	64	138	18.0

This includes nonexistent or unverifiable journals/articles/books/papers, abstract but not a manuscript, "in press" but never appeared, and inaccuracy in position in authorship.

authors of a long list of authors is probably important, being the last author or near last author in a long list is also probably important, being in the middle of a large group of authors means very little, and there is no real convention in authorship listing.

- *Encourage your group to include a "Contributions" section in the paper.* This can include those people involved in some capacity, but whose real contribution does not warrant authorship.
- *Stick to the numbers – develop a point system.* You should create a grading/point system for each contribution that was made to the study based on its intensity and importance.
- *Be picky about who you work with – good and poor collaborators* (pay attention to "reputations"). There are some lab directors who are known for their insistence on being mentioned as authors in every single paper. I know an individual who opened a lab in another country, brought in funds, built a team, and started collecting data. His notion was, "This is my lab. You work for me. My name needs to be mentioned in every single manuscript that comes from here regardless of my effort on the actual project." This is called a reputation. Do you want to work for someone like this? Some mentors don't trust students to write the first draft and prefer to write it themselves to get it done quicker. This means that the students end up graduating with no experience in writing. If the student gets credit for the work regardless, for example, first authorship, this is not doing the student any favors. This, in fact, could cause major problems as the student will be expected to be proficient at writing and publishing papers by future employers.

To resolve any disputes if they may arise, I recommend the following:

- *Find the happy medium – share work and credit.* It usually feels good when you share both work and credit as deserved.
- *Get professional advice – mentors.* You will always need a mentor no matter how old you get or how much experience you gain.
- *Keep good records.* Keep track of all meetings/emails/phone logs as you never know when you may need to use them if any disputes will arise.
- *Keep your cool – be civil and DO NOT behave badly.* You will not gain anything if you have a confrontation, and you certainly do not want to burn any bridges.

5.3.7   Authorship stories

Before we move away from the topic of authorship, I would like to give you some "nightmare" stories in order to help you fully comprehend how horrible such a situation could become if we do not control it (Vignettes 5.6 and 5.7). You can find many additional scenarios at: http://ori.hhs.gov/ education/products/niu_authorship/mistakes/index.htm

I believe you should take public responsibility for the work that you publish, not just the credit from it. If you are a coauthor on a manuscript, then you had better be aware of everything that is mentioned in the paper. I have 30 publications from collaborators overseas. I used to travel to these foreign laboratories three times a year. I used to spend a week on each visit. During those visits, I attended many data collections (that I had also designed myself) to make sure everything was flawless. I taught the researchers how to digitize the data and gave them my own programs

---

**VIGNETTE 5.6   Pressure from the top
(from personal communication)**

Let's say you have just taken a relatively junior position in a very well-established research group at a new institution. A few months later, as you are preparing a paper for publication in *Nature* based mostly on work from your previous location, you ask the well-known section chief to review the paper prior to journal submission. The chief carefully reads the paper and makes many critical or constructive comments. You also notice that the chief has added his/her name to the author list and in a final note volunteers to cover the page charges if the article is accepted. *What do you do?*

- Would you include the "chief" who reviewed your paper and will pay for the page costs as an author?
- What are the options?
- How can you justify adding him/her as an author?
- Is including him/her as author scientific misconduct?

Based on JAMA's criteria, the chief does not have the right to be included as a coauthor. Based solely on the first criterion, for example, he/she neither conceived nor designed the study or made a "substantial contribution" to the acquisition, analysis, or interpretation of the data. Unfortunately, this case is a real one. The chief created a tremendous amount of stress for the author since he/she was the boss. This led to a huge conflict between the two individuals and the situation escalated leading to the young faculty member having to leave. It is crucial to consider very carefully the people you might work with.

VIGNETTE 5.7   Mr. Hard Cell (Hooper, 2006)

A highly respected scientist in Korea made significant progress in a controversial research area dealing with embryonic
stem cells and cloning. He was promptly joined by a shrewd
American scientist on a major study that was anticipated to
lead to groundbreaking results, publication and a great deal
of public visibility. The American collaborator aided in the
study design, acted as a sounding board for the project and
helped troubleshoot problems as they arose, but did not play
any role in the bench research undertaken at the Korean lab.
The results of the study were published in *Science* where
they were both authors. The headlines went global and there
was much celebration. Later, the Korean scientist is accused
of improprieties related to how he sought egg donors for the
stem cell research projects and data fabrication. Specifically,
he was discovered to have pressured his junior staff – female
technicians and postdoctoral students – into donating! The
American scientist asked the journal *Science* for his name to be
withdrawn as an author of the high-profile paper. The journal
refused. The Korean scientist is later accused of fraud, embez-
zlement and bioethics violations that were related not only to
the *Science* publication but to other projects as well. Ultimately,
the Korean scientist is found to be guilty of misconduct and
lost his job and reputation. The papers are withdrawn. Did
the American investigator who was also an author on the
paper commit scientific misconduct? Why or why not? What
should be the consequences for the American investigator?
"Dr. Gerald Schatten was found to have demonstrated a 'lack
of judgement' and participated in 'research misbehavior' but
not scientific misconduct (Hooper, 2006)." Dr. Schatten does
have his job, he is not in jail, yet he has his name (and often
his face) plastered across many presentations about scientific
misconduct.

---

to process the data. After attaining the data, I reanalyzed the data many
times to make sure the results were accurate. If I uncovered issues, I asked
for the initial raw data so that I could reprocess it and make sure no errors
were present. I also ran all statistical analyses myself or used my Omaha-
based biostatistician. Lastly, I asked my collaborators to write the first
draft, which I always read carefully and usually revised extensively. How
confident was I in the data? I was extremely confident.

5.4 Plagiarism

According to the *Merriam-Webster* dictionary, plagiarism originates from the Latin word *plagiarius*, which means "someone that steals the words of another." Plagiarism is essentially presenting, as one's own, an idea or product derived from an existing source. It also occurs in science. In a very interesting international case, a scientist from Iraq published 60 articles as if they were his own by stealing them from small obscure journals (Henderson, 1990).

I do not want to devote too much space on plagiarism and research misconduct, as everybody knows what it is and is very well aware of it. However, I do want to mention a few remedies. First, always cite the references you use. Second, if you are using some text verbatim, use quotation marks. Third, specify sections of cited publications for any paraphrased text. Fourth, be aware of copyright restrictions for images. Fifth, you can self-plagiarize but again watch out for copyright restrictions. Lastly, and this is more for my international students, challenges of language and writing skill, or respect for an expert's opinion, do not validate copying without proper acknowledgement.

5.5 The peer-review process

This is a topic that was not found frequently under academic ethics. However, I consider it as a very important topic because reviewers also need to take their responsibilities very seriously and conduct their reviews with the highest ethical manner. Personal or any other type of bias does not have any place in the reviewing process. I tremendously appreciate the fact that I have to sign a CONFLICT OF INTEREST, CONFIDENTIALITY, AND NON-DISCLOSURE form when I review for the NIH, the Department of Veterans Affairs (VA), and many other agencies. I am also pleased to see now days the utilization of such forms by academic journals.

Every time that I review, I always remember the quote below from my good friend Dr. Howard Zelaznik. I think this is the best advice a scientist can get when reviewing manuscripts and grants.

> Do not evaluate research based on how you would have conducted a study; judge the work on its own merits. This simple principle has allowed me to try to search for good in each experiment and study. This principle does not mean that I recommend acceptance of every paper, but it does prevent me from being overly critical about the manner in which the experiment was not done (i.e. the experiment was not conducted "my way").

> *(Zelaznik, 1993, page 66)*

I have actually copied this quote and placed it on my desk to remind me of it every time I review a paper. In addition to this quote, I have also included below some tips on how to be an effective reviewer.

1. Try to provide constructive criticism and don't be vague.
2. Be cordial and polite.
3. Never appraise the work based on how YOU would do this study, but always assess the study on its own merits.
4. Only review studies in areas that you are knowledgeable about.
5. Maintain a database of all your reviews. You will find yourself repeating comments many times.
6. Create a template and use it every time.
7. If you really believe that the paper doesn't have a chance to be accepted, reject it. Still provide constructive criticism. This will eliminate time with multiple revisions.
8. Don't be an editor (trying to teach someone how to write a paper) but a scientific reviewer.

In Vignette 5.8, I have provided an example on what I consider an effective review of a manuscript.

VIGNETTE 5.8   An example of an effective review

COMMENTS TO THE EDITOR

Thank you very much for allowing me the opportunity to review this manuscript. I truly believe the results of the study are relevant to your readers. However, I have serious concerns as to how the data are presented (or rather lack thereof). The authors fail to present actual data regarding demographic information of the study cohort, medians and ranges of outcomes, and p values. I have tried to provide suggestions as to how they can improve the manuscript. I would be more than happy to re-review this manuscript once the changes are made.

COMMENTS TO THE AUTHORS

1 GENERAL COMMENTS

The authors present an interesting study. Remodeling of graft material after anterior cruciate ligament (ACL) reconstruction with regard to the so-called ligamentization is of great importance for determining rehabilitation protocols and return to sports guidelines. Although this subject has been studied in animal studies, it has not been extensively studied in humans. There are similar studies published on the topic, but I still believe this work to be of importance to the readers of this journal. The length of the manuscript is appropriate and it is generally well written.

2 INTRODUCTION

The introduction provides adequate background. The purpose is clear.

- Please provide a hypothesis for your study.
- Line 31: ... postoperatively. This sentence needs a reference.
- Line 38 ... compare to animal studies. Your reference does not support this statement. The referred study is a human study only.
- I am a little bit concerned because the references used by the authors are older and although they are important, newer work should be referenced too in the introduction. Please see reference section for some suggestions.

3 METHODS (MATERIAL, PATIENTS, AND METHODS)

The method section is clear. The surgical technique is adequately described, as is the histological analysis. Information about the study cohort is lacking. Please provide the age, sex, etc. of your studied population. If available, activity level would be useful, that is, were they competitive athletes, recreational athletes, or sedentary individuals.

- Line 12: please report all reasons for second look arthroscopy and their distribution.
- Line 56: please provide a reference for this standardized accelerated rehabilitation protocol you refer to, or describe it briefly, since many different ones exist.
- Line 58: please clarify "sports participation." Is this full return to competitive contact sports? Or just level jogging, etc.
- Line 10: please explain how these three different time groups were chosen.
- Line 12: please explain how native ACL specimens were obtained and how many were used. Was this from the same subjects?

- Statistical analysis is appropriate. However, in the case of Mann–Whitney if multiple comparisons are made (in this case three groups which means three comparisons), the Bonferroni correction should be applied, correcting the p value for the number of comparisons. So, for the results of the Mann–Whitney test alpha should be set as $<0.05/3 = <0.02$.

4 RESULTS

The results are very interesting, but the results section needs some work. There are two few major issues:

1. There is no demographic information of your studied population. Therefore, the homogeneity of your subjects cannot be determined. Since you do not follow subjects over time, but rather classify biopsies from individual subjects in different time frames, this information is very important. You aim to create a "time line" of changes within the ACL graft suggestive of healing/ligamentization, but strictly with your study design this cannot be done. You would need sequential biopsies from the same subjects to definitively conclude this. However, it is understood this is difficult to execute. Therefore, the reliability of your time line created from individual subjects is based on the homogeneity of these subjects. This includes age, sex, median, and range of the time after surgery when the biopsy was done, reasons for second look, number of subjects in each of the three groups, and number of native ACLs. If you provide this information, your study would be much better to interpret.

2. The results are not adequately reported. Only the median values of the cell counts is reported, but also the range should be reported (or mean and standard deviation). When reporting an increase or decrease in cell count, you need to state if this is a "significant" increase (and report the p value) or if it is just a visible trend (in which case I would opt not to report it at all). It would also be better to report the two medians or means between which there is an increase of decrease. For example, the cell count between groups 1 and 2 significantly increased from 1,000,000 to 1,500,000 ($p = 0.03$). Your figures are very

valuable in this, but the significance needs to be shown appropriately in your figures with * and *p* value, and explained in the figure legend.

More specific concerns are addressed below:

- Line 9: "Compared to native HT, there was a significant difference to group 1 ($p \leq 0.05$)" Please rephrase this to clarify. Was there no difference between groups 2 and 3 and the native HT? It does look like there should be in table 1 and figure 1. As implied by "Total cell number was increased in all groups...." The *p* value here is missing. Please report the exact *p* value, for example, $p = 0.041$, not $p < 0.05$.
- Line 15: "The cell number decreased from group 2 to 3 without reaching the cell density level of the native ACL" was this difference significant? If so, please report the *p* value. If this is just a visible trend from the graph, you cannot state there is a decrease.
- Lines 17–27: "Vessel density showed the lowest value in group 1 where it was also decreased compared to both controls. Consecutively, vessel density increased up to the level of native HT in group 2 and higher values in group 3 without reaching the vessel density of the ACL at any time point. Compared to ACLs, native HT had a significantly lower vessel density." Were all these changes significant? Then all of these statements need *p* values. Please refer to the previous comment.
- Lines 29–37: "Myofibroblast density was higher in all groups compared to native controls with significant higher values in group 2 compared to native HT ($p = 0.045$) and it increased clearly from group 1 to 2. From group 2 to 3, myofibroblast density decreased but was still clearly increased compared to native controls." Same concern: were all these changes significant? If so, *p* values need to be reported for all of them individually.

5 DISCUSSION

The discussion section is interesting and generally well written. However, please start the section with the sentence: The most important finding of this study was...

Adequate comparisons with existing literature are made. However, I would suggest that rather than first discussing all existing literature and then their own findings, the authors individually compare the discussed literature to their own findings. For example, xxx et al. found that …. However, our study showed …. yyy et al. found that …. Our study also showed this…. Structuring the discussion section like that would make it easier to read.

As mentioned before, there is some concern about the publication date of the references, most are very old. Please see reference section for suggestions.

A significant limitation of the study that needs to be discussed in that the biopsy samples were used to create a "time line" for ACL graft remodeling; the samples were not taken at subsequent time from the same individuals, but belonged to different individuals. (See previous comment in the results.) Therefore, care should be taken to conclude that changes occur in the graft from one time point to another, since this cannot be verified in the same subjects and may therefore be partially attributed to amongst-subject variation.

A positive point of your study is that – although non-anatomical – your reconstructive procedure was consistent, done by one surgeon and with one graft type, providing a homogeneous subset, as appropriately acknowledged in the discussion.

- Line 15: … their own findings. This sentence needs a reference.

6 CONCLUSION

The conclusion is more an extended discussion. Please try to conclude only the major findings of your study, without comparisons to what is known, or future directives.

7 ABSTRACT

The abstract is well written. It could be shortened. In the results section, please report actual results, such as cell count, in numbers, and exact p values.

8 TITLE

The title is not appropriate and should be modified. The segment "analysis over 10 years" should be removed, as it implies that patients were followed for 10 years, or biopsies were taken over a 10-year time frame within the same patients, which is not the case. I would suggest: Remodeling of hamstring autografts after ACL reconstruction or Remodeling of hamstring autografts after ACL reconstruction: a histological analysis.

9 REFERENCES

The references are not up to date; there is only one reference for 2009–2010. Recent references should be added. Please find a few relevant ones below. The used references are adequate and should be kept, if new ones are added. Please check that the issue number is missing in some references. Otherwise, the format looks appropriate.

10 FIGURES

The figures are appropriate and should be kept. However, the figure legend is insufficient. It is unclear what the big bar, middle bar and long bars are: Mean? Median? Standard deviation? Range? 95% Confidence interval? What marks significance? And between which bars does the significance occur?

- Figure 2: the y-axis scale should be changed to better fit the bars. There is unused space, while the bars appear very small.
- Figure 3: same as figure 2.
- Figure 4 is really helpful. It would be nice if an example of group 2 can be added.
- Figure 5: same as figure 4.

11 TABLES

Table 1 is useful. However, only median is reported, but there is no range given. Please add range. Another suggestion would be to report overall p values of the Kruskall Wallis in the table, so the readers can see which variables change from group 1 to 3. However, this is merely a suggestion and the authors should make this decision. In my opinion, it would most likely improve the readability of the manuscript.

5.6   *Mentoring and advising*

Mentorship and advising is also a large part of my work as a scientist and is also one that is often vulnerable to misconduct. Mentoring is fundamental for your scientific career, regardless of whether you stay in academia or venture beyond. Especially in academia, I believe that everyone is mentoring and being mentored; doctoral students might be mentoring other graduate students or undergraduates, graduate students are mentoring undergraduates, senior undergraduates are mentoring junior undergraduates, junior faculty are mentoring several graduate students (postdocs, doctoral students, and master students), senior faculty are mentoring junior faculty, etc. You may not even have to be present to mentor someone. I still have a mentor even at my academic level of a Dean. Mentorship is performed daily in our lives, as it is part of our profession, and it is extremely important.

5.6.1   Origins of a historical mentor

Homer's epic poem, *The Odyssey*, was written in about 900 BC. The lead character, Odysseus, Greek King of the Island Ithaca, left to fight in the Trojan War leaving his wife, Penelope, and son, Telemachus, in Ithaca. The goddess of wisdom, Athena, cared for Odysseus and took on the form of *Mentor* (was also called as such) to guide and counsel Telemachus in his father's absence. Odysseus was gone for 20 years and when he came back he found that Mentor had faithfully guided his son to become an intelligent, ambitious, and wise young man (Figures 5.1 and 5.2). Here are a few words from Odyssey:

Telemachus: Mentor, how am I to go up to the great man? How shall I greet him? Remember that I have no practice in making speeches; and a young man may well hesitate to cross-examine one so much his senior.

Mentor: Telemachus, where your native wit fails, heaven will inspire you. It is not for nothing that the gods have watched your progress ever since your birth.[1]

Based on the above, the characteristics of the (historical) mentor are as follows:

- Wise in all things
- Caring for the Protégé
- Protective of his/her charge
- Persistent in his/her task
- Powerful beyond belief
- A Greek Goddess/God in disguise[2]

---

[1] Most graduate students feel shy when first presenting or teaching because they have not had much practice in public speaking. I remember when I was young, and I had my first meeting with one of the most famous biomechanists, Dr. Walter Herzog, and I was sweating. Similarly, couple of years ago, a young graduate student was going through the same thing when he first met me!

[2] One of the historical mentor's characteristics is being a Greek God/Goddess in disguise. My doctoral student and now Dr. Jenny Kent always jokes that this is the reason that she came to be mentored by me!

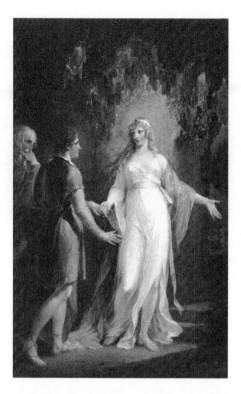

Figure 5.1 Calypso receiving Telemachus and Mentor in the Grotto (William Hamilton, 1785). This painting depicts the meeting that took place between Telemachus and the nymph Calypso, on Telemachus' search for his father, Odysseus. Athena, as Mentor, is standing behind Telemachus to observe and provide advice if needed.

5.6.2 What mentors really do?

Advise, counsel, and inform. As a senior faculty that mentors junior faculty, I need to provide them with information that will help their careers. I might inform them about agencies where they can apply for grants and even courses that they need to teach. I may even suggest courses for them to improve their knowledge in specific areas, ultimately helping their careers (you never stop learning). In terms of advice and counsel, you can provide not only encouragement but also constructive criticism.[3] We should appreciate the mentors that provide genuine advice and criticism that will ensure success instead of just motivating and encouraging their mentees. During

---

[3] Even your parents shouldn't pat you on your back all the time. My mom did not pat me on my back all the time but many times gave me tough love!

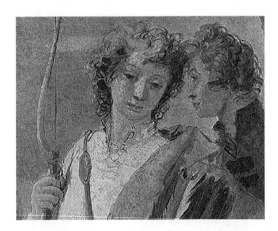

Figure 5.2 Telemachus and Mentor (Giovanni Battista Tiepolo, 1740). This painting also shows Telemachus with Mentor standing behind him, whispering in his ear words of advice and council if needed.

my early PhD years at the University of Oregon, my mentor Dr. Barry Bates was giving a lecture on shoe design, and even though I had knowledge of the literature on that topic, I was still naïve. I remember during that lecture, I opposed one of his comments, providing evidence from a specific paper. Little did I know, the paper I quoted was performed in a completely inaccurate manner. Dr. Bates responded by saying "Nick with you, we have to de-educate you, and then re-educate you again." His comment was based on the fact that I couldn't identify the faults in that paper I was citing. Another time I asked him about my level compared to other PhD students he had, and he just smiled and replied, "just work hard!"

Share career experiences. I teach a course every year that I call "The mistakes that Dr. Stergiou made in Academia and how to avoid them!" This course is full of personal experiences, and I have shared numerous such experiences with you throughout this book.

Support (emotional, moral, financial). Sometimes we might face a downturn, and we might need emotional, moral, and financial support. Back when I was a graduate student, I did not have money to travel back home at Christmas, so my mentor paid for my ticket so I could travel and see my family.

Give feedback; acknowledge accomplishments. It is very important to acknowledge the accomplishments of your mentees. Give them credit in front of others when they deserve it.

Give time; listen. Many times, your mentees just need a sounding board.

Help establish goals; respect those goals. This is extremely important as young people don't know how to develop goals. This is also seen in senior people.

Challenge and encourage ... be positive. This means that you, as a mentor, need to challenge your mentee to make them better. For example, in Greek mythology, when Aegeus (who gave his name to the Aegean Sea) left his son Theseus to become the King of Athens, Theseus asked him why he was not taking him along. His father told him that he was not yet ready. He said that when Theseus was able to push a huge rock and retrieve Aegeus' sword from under it, then he could come to him and bring him his sword. That was a challenge that Aegeus provided to his son, along with a demand for consistent training with isometric muscular contractions!

Promote or sponsor; help with networking. We invite several brilliant scientists from around the globe to UNO, and I always encourage our faculty and students to meet them and introduce themselves to enhance networking.

Serve as an academic/clinical model. How can you expect your mentees to perform their jobs and work hard if you are an apathetic mentor? If you are not the person to look up to? Alexander the Great is one of the most well-known, well-respected leaders. He convinced 40,000 people to practically walk from Greece to India, while carrying heavy armor in a war zone while fighting enemies. During that time, medical care was undeveloped, and people had to close their wounds using fire and other techniques. People were dying from minor injuries. How did he accomplish such a feat? He was a true leader. Once they were crossing a desert and had run out of water. He sent scouts ahead to find water. When they found a source, they brought some water back and gave it to him. He emptied the bottle in front of all his soldiers and said, "I will drink when everybody else drinks".

Improve the apprentice/protégé; teach. You should aim for your mentee to leave as your equal, or even better than you.

Continue mentoring after degree is completed. Mentorship is a lifetime job. I still seek advice and mentorship from Dr. Bates to this day, and he is still harsh with me.

5.6.3 Myths about mentoring

Here are what I call myths about mentoring:

The best way to succeed is to have a mentor. It is important to have a mentor, but it is not necessary. Similarly, you could have a great mentor but not succeed because you don't listen to him or her.

Mentoring is always beneficial. We could put ourselves in a detrimental situation if we don't choose our mentors carefully.

The mentor should be older. A mentor can be young and can be younger than you. I still have PhD students that I have a strong relationship with, who are older than me.

A person can have only one mentor at a time. You can have multiple, simultaneous mentors from whom you seek advice.

Mentoring is all for the benefit of the protégé. The mentor also receives great benefits if the protégé performs great work and does a great job. That is also fulfilling for the mentor. That is why mentoring is truly amazing.

If you are seeking a mentor, wait to be asked. We should seek the mentor instead of the mentor seeking us.

Men are better mentors for women. Gender has no effect on mentorship. One of my mentors is a female working at the University of Texas at Austin, Dr. Jody Jensen.

The mentor always knows best. The mentor provides advice and does not set the law.

Anyone can be a mentor. Several people cannot become a mentor because they can't set an example or provide advice, because they do not have the experience necessary, because they do not work well with others, or because they find it hard to allocate time to nurture their students' development.

5.6.4   How do you become a good mentor?

Below are some advices on how to become a good mentor.

Hire good people that love to work hard (if you love to work hard). As you have read already, my favorite motto is "I may not be able to outsmart anyone, but I can outwork everybody." The students who come to me need to be hardworking; otherwise, our habits won't match. It works both ways. I work well with my current doctoral student, Jenny Kent, as we are both hard workers and want the best. I would be a terrible mentor for her if I didn't work hard. How about if the mentee is extremely smart but does not want to work? This depends on what the mentor is looking for, but that will still be an unhealthy relationship. Even the smartest people cannot accomplish anything without committing to the work.

Be sacrificial and nurture their development. You sacrifice time, effort, emotion, even money sometimes. Remember that what a student wants aren't necessarily what is best for them. Care for your students' personal lives as well as their careers. Be invested. Put them first. Push them so they can understand their limits[4].

---

[4] My mentor had an interesting style of mentoring. I used to ask him for work, and he used to provide it until it got to the point that I couldn't take it anymore. I then had to go to him to ask him to reduce my workload. "Ha!" he said. "So, you've finally realized that you cannot do it all?" That was such a great lesson. He kept doing that with all his students. He would force you to the edge, and then when you realized that you couldn't do everything at the same time, he would start taking things from you. It's a very humbling experience.

Have an open door policy to the best of your ability. I always keep my door open, and when I am there my students know they can come in and talk to me.

Spend time with them through Reading Clubs and seminars. One of the best ways to nurture the development of your students is through Reading Clubs. It is the best course you can have as a graduate student. Being able to read and critique articles with others is one of the best ways of generating ideas and developing your abilities as a scientist (see also chapter one).

Aim for your mentee to leave as your equal. Or even better than you, if possible. I frequently direct questions I get asked to my previous students who are now experts in specific fields, instead of trying to answer them myself. My students know more than me in those areas.

Never let an email go unanswered. You never know who will be contacting you. It could be someone from Greece (like me) who wants to come and join your graduate education! Someone answered my inquiry a long time ago, and I got the greatest gift of all time – to become a scientist.

Work harder than them so you can lead by example. If they give you 10 h of work, try to do 11.

Have social events to improve collegiality. Different mentors have different approaches here – some mentors encourage it and others don't. Younger mentors often tend to be more social, and more senior faculty less so. I particularly like the occasional drink with my students.

You want their respect but not their love. You want your mentees to respect you. Otherwise, why would they think they can learn from you?

5.6.5 How can you be a good mentee?

Below is some advice on how to be a good mentee.

Match your mentor's work ethic. If you don't like to work on the weekends, make sure they are not the kind of person that does. I remember a potential postdoc who could not commit to writing a short weekly report over the weekend because his philosophy was "I do not work during the weekend." He ended up not joining my research team.

Cultivate a relationship. The relationship between mentor and mentee is considered as strong as your relationship with your parents. I remember when I got married, my mentor, Dr. Barry Bates stepped in on behalf of my father during the wedding since I do not have a father.

Leave your ego at the door. Watch how Master Miyaki molds Karate Kid by having him paint the fence in the original movie. What a classic example! Trust and accept authority. How would you expect to have a healthy relationship with your mentor if you don't listen to him/her? You must trust your mentor and listen to advice when you are provided with it.

5.6.6   *Finding good mentors*

There are environments in which you will not have time to talk to your mentor because he/she is very busy. There are environments where your mentor could give you back your paper after 6 months without any feedback. There are environments within which the mentors will write all the papers with their name as first author. There are environments within which you will not be allowed to write your own grants just because they want you to start working on their experiments. These are environments you want to avoid.

So, what are the rules for finding good Mentors?

1. Seek them out. Know their work; make sure they have expertise in your area of interest.
2. Conduct auditions. You must conduct auditions in the same way that you would conduct dates when looking for your significant other. Ask important questions such as: What is it like in the lab? Could I thrive there?
3. Talk to their current and past students. Talk to them!
4. How often should you expect to meet with them? What should you expect from them, and what are you expected to give? [5]
5. Do they provide opportunities outside research? For example, do they fund conference travel or provide assistance with international travel?
6. Do they actually care for their students? You may be able to gauge this by talking to the prospective mentor, but it may be more reliable to actually visit their laboratory to witness how they interact with their students, and to ask the mentor's previous students for their opinion.

5.6.7   *Ethics in mentoring and advising of graduate students*

A very influential paper I have read regarding ethics in mentoring and advising of graduate students is written by Roberts in 1993. Here, I would like to take a closer look at some quotes from this article. This paper may seem more relevant to mentors (young and senior professors) as they advise their graduate students, but it will also be relevant to mentees as they in turn become mentors and face the same ethical issues (Roberts, 1993).

---

[5] When I was looking for a university for my PhD, for example, I realized that one of the mentors I was looking into working with would not be able to provide time to meet and interact with me on a regular basis. I wouldn't have known this if I hadn't taken the time to talk to him and find out about him from his students.

The best advisors, however, have the welfare of the student at heart and attempt to attend to both aspects of adequate supervision of graduate students. The first and most important has to do with creativity and involves the ability to select problems, to stimulate and enthuse students, and to provide a steady stream of ideas for student to digest.

The most crucial and impactful factor, on which a good advisor needs to focus his/her attention when mentoring a graduate student, is nurturing their independent problem solving and creative abilities. If the advisor is not capable of providing these features, then you, as a student, must find another mentor. A scientist must to be able to generate ideas, as it is the most important skill in this profession. Generating ideas should be part of the learning process and discussed in class, reading clubs, meetings, and even at lunch (see chapter one). The scientific "investigative" ability needs to be cultivated by the mentor, especially at the doctoral level. This can only be achieved through intensive reading, scientific discussion, attending stimulating classes, and even a specific style of advising.

The advisor does great harm who uses the student simply as a technician on a piece of equipment, a "data cruncher," or a convenient research "instrument." The student is supposed to be learning to contribute to knowledge, especially in the dissertation; therefore, we should not expect less from any student during the rest of the program. We are in the business of developing productive scholars, not efficient technicians. We do not help our students by expecting less. We are ethically bound to produce scholars who will go on to make their own professional contributions.

I do know many advisors who are themselves great technicians and produce great student technicians but have made limited contributions to science. The field of Biomechanics has many of these scientists, and those who practice true scholarly activities are in such short supply. As graduate students, you live an extremely stressful life, and you don't get much financial support, because you want to dedicate your entire time and effort to science. Thus, you must pursue a PhD that will guide you to become an extremely good scholar; a "Sherlock Holmes" of science.

A unique and special relationship exists between the PhD student and her or his advisor. They start as master and apprentice and ideally end up as colleagues.

Developing colleagues should be the goal of every advisor instead of developing apprentices.

> When we discuss quality programs in our field...
> we tend to focus on two criteria of excellence. One
> pertains to the quality of students as they enter
> programs, the other to the quality of the faculty at
> a particular institution. ... the assumption under-
> lying student entrance and continuation criteria
> is that excellent scholars will emerge if we have
> excellent students to begin with. But rigorous
> entrance requirements do not guarantee excellent
> scholars. Entrance constraints are necessary but not
> sufficient for postdoctoral success.

If you have a perfect GRE score, TOFEL, and GPA, it doesn't mean that you will be a perfect scholar or a great doctoral student. When I was in Oregon, we had a student that had perfect scores in addition to being artistic. My mentor had great hopes for him. He left within a year, as he wasn't able to concentrate, apply himself, or work hard enough. Entrance requirements are important and should be considered, but they are not everything. Determination is extremely important.

> To determine the antecedents of Nobel awards,
> Zuckerman analyzed the education of the 92 Nobel
> Prize winners of the United States until 1972. The
> first relationship noted is that over 50% of Nobel
> Prize winners had worked with Nobel laure-
> ates either as graduate students or in postdoctoral
> positions.

Excellence breeds excellence. It's as simple as that.

> The distinguishing characteristic of these effective
> mentors was their emphasis on the process of being
> a scholar. At the heart of this role modeling is the
> necessity for the faculty member to spend time with
> the student. A consistent complaint of doctoral stu-
> dents is that time with them – not only in research
> advising but also in professional advising and
> discourse.

Although this paper was published more than 20 years ago, it discusses issues we still face today. I know several advisors who take months to provide feedback on students' papers. At that time, before the internet was introduced, scientists relied on physical proximity (e.g. meetings) for opportunities to discuss work. Nowadays scientists can easily work from any location. There should be no reason not to reply to your students, regardless of the time and place. Students should always receive the attention they need and deserve. If my PhD student sends me an email, I reply as soon as possible. If I receive a paper to review from my student, I try to respond within a few days. In Vignette 5.9, I have also listed some good advising practices as provided by the Council of Graduate Schools.

VIGNETTE 5.9   Good graduate advising practice (Council of Graduate Schools, 1990)

1. Involve the student in all phases of the research process.

    The mentor should involve his/her students in every aspect of research; writing grants, data collections, data analysis, and writing the paper.
2. Encourage students to develop their own research agendas.

    Ask your students to develop their own logical tree. One of our demands for first year PhD students is to write and submit a grant. When students write a grant, they have to think about the aims, develop a research question, and build a methodology. After the grant is submitted, they are provided with feedback from the reviewers. I am in favor of providing grant writing exercises for doctoral students. In my opinion, it is the best exercise for graduate students.
3. Read their work in a reasonable time.

    You must prioritize reading your students' papers and provide feedback within a week.
4. Read materials with a critical eye, offering ample suggestions and comments.

    Try to provide meaningful comments to your students if any are needed.
5. Be accessible and be prepared to discuss all aspects of professional endeavor.

    In our times, if you receive an email, answer it as soon as possible.
6. Be someone who knows her or his own mind, makes a decision, and sticks to it.

    This is difficult scientifically; you tend to change your mind frequently as a scientist. When advising, it is important to be consistent in what you ask of your student, though. During my PhD, for example, Dr. Bates asked me to take Lagrangian mechanics. It was the first

---

time I had heard of it, and I haven't used it since, except
when I reviewed a couple of papers that used the techniques. I tried every method I could to convince Dr. Bates
to let me withdraw from the course. But I couldn't, as he
refused to change his decision and ordered me to take the
course as every other student had had to take it. Maybe
that's what this point is about.

7. Never allow a student to become "cannon fodder" in a
dispute with a colleague.

Back in Oregon, there was a doctoral student who
never cleaned up after his data collections and used up
a load of data space on the server. I was in charge of data
storage, and my duty was to make sure that the server
was always empty for data collection. We had to move
all the data to magnetic tapes for storage. His inability
to do this almost caused a major dispute between us.
I complained to our mentor, and he resolved the issue
by talking to the doctoral student while preventing me
from making any irrational decisions. Always try to
calm your student in order to find a rational solution.
It is necessary to promote discussions among students
(maybe during team meetings), but the mentor must
provide guidance and time for these issues as they are
critical.

8. Keep the relationship with the student strictly professional.

I think the word "strictly" is too harsh, but the relationship must be kept professional. During my master's
degree, my mentors and I would go out for drinks every
Friday. I was once invited to a mentor's beach house.
During my PhD, Dr. Bates was completely different. On
the other hand, as a mentor, I used to spend a lot of time
with my students socially during my early career. Now
that I am older, I try not to do that, so I won't blur the
lines.

9. Monitor professional progress.

Our PhD students are required to maintain a portfolio of their work every year in order to do this. During
my PhD, and here at UNO before we established our
Biomechanics department, we used to ask the PhD students to update their CVs every year.

References

American Psychological Association Ethics Committee. (1983). *Authorship Guidelines for Dissertation Supervision*. Washington, DC.

Bates, T., Anić, A., Marušić, M., Marušić, A. (2004). Authorship criteria and disclosure of contributions: comparison of 3 general medical journals with different author contribution forms. *JAMA*, 292(1), 86–88.

Chang, K. (2010). Nobel Laureate Retracts Two Papers Unrelated to Her Prize. *The New York Times*, September 23.

Council of Graduate Schools. (1990). *Research Student and Supervisor: An Approach to Good Supervisory Practice*. Washington, DC.

Daniels, P.S. (1985). Author retraction. *Psychophysiology*, 22, 217.

Fine, M.A., Kurdek, L.A. (1993). Reflections on determining authorship credit and authorship order on faculty-student collaborations. *American Psychologist*, 48(11), 1141–1147.

Harris, G. (2009). Doctor Admits Pain Studies Were Frauds, Hospital Says. *The New York Times*, March 11.

Henderson, J. (1990). When scientists fake it. *American Way*, 56–62, 100–101.

Hooper, J. (2006). Mr Hard Cell. *Popular Science*, 269(2), 64–91.

Landers, D.M., Christina, R.S. (1986). Notice. *Journal of Sport Psychology*, 8, 144.

Office of Science and Technology Policy. (2000). Final federal policy on research misconduct. *The Federal Register*, 65(235), 76260–762641.

Roberts, G.C. (1993). Ethics in professional advising and academic counseling of graduate students. *Quest*, 45(1), 78–87.

Wade, N. (2010). Harvard Finds Marc Hauser Guilty of Scientific Misconduct. *The New York Times*, August 20.

Wilcox, L.J. (1998). Authorship: the coin of the realm, the source of complaints. *JAMA*, 280(3), 216–217.

Wilmore, J.H. (1979). Letter to the editor. Medicine and Science in Sports, H, iii.

Zelaznik, H.N. (1993). Ethical issues in conducting and reporting research: a reaction to Kroll, Matt, and Safrit. *Quest*, 45(1), 62–68.

chapter six

Management and organization

Learning never exhausts the mind.

—Leonardo da Vinci (1452–1519)

6.1 Introduction

This chapter discusses a number of important skills regarding time and laboratory management and organization that are needed in order to become a successful scientist and academician. However, many of these skills, and my corresponding advice, also apply to employment in the industry and life, in general. For example, knowing how to effectively manage your time is an issue that stresses almost everybody in our modern societies.

6.2 Time management

Almost every person in academia (students, junior, and even senior faculty), along with professionals in other fields, struggles with time management. All of my previous PhD students have reached out to me at some point to find a solution for their time management problems. I consider poor planning, personal disorganization, and procrastination, the three big killers of productivity, and my time management techniques are geared towards defeating them.

To start, I consider the following as my ten "commandments" of time management:

1. Identify how you spend your time.
2. Recognize when your productivity is at a maximum.
3. Plan tomorrow's work today.
4. Consider the reason for performing every task in your agenda.
5. Deal with each piece of information you receive (email, file, etc.) once.
6. Plan your work, but also make sure that you work according to your plan.
7. Delegate prudently.

8. Prioritize your tasks.
9. Learn to delete and maintain cleanliness.
10. Recognize the importance of your tasks.

Below I will try to further emphasize some of these commandments.

6.2.1   Be proactive

> I have two kinds of problems, the urgent and the important. The urgent are not important, and the important are never urgent.
>
> *(Dwight D. Eisenhower, 1890–1969)*

Your tasks as an academic (graduate student, research associate, technician, faculty member, etc.) vary from those that are work related (write grants, teach courses, attend classes, prepare exams, grade exams, take exams, write papers, etc.) to those from your personal life (cook for your children, buy groceries, do laundry, etc.). All of your tasks can be organized into one of the four quadrants of this schematic below (Figure 6.1), which will guide their prioritization. This is known as the Eisenhower method (see the quote above).

Here are some examples so we can understand these different quadrants.

Urgent and important tasks: A grant deadline will be such a task, especially if you need the funds to support your laboratory or if your promotion relies on it.

Not urgent and important tasks: Writing a grant with a deadline 4 months is such a task. Writing a paper that could be important for your promotion that is due in several months is another such task.

Urgent but not important tasks: Picking up your clothes from the dry-cleaning shop at a specific date they have provided is a typical

	URGENT	NOT URGENT
IMPORTANT	Necessity	Proactive
NOT IMPORTANT	Comfort	Trivia

Figure 6.1 Four quadrants that designate the level of importance to the task.

example of this type of task. Other personal tasks could be urgent where the deadline is imminent but the task itself is not as important.

Not urgent and not important tasks: Checking your spam email folder will be such a task.

Cleaning up your desk before you leave is Proactive Thinking. Cleaning it in the morning is Comfort Thinking. Spending a lot of time googling the best way of cleaning it is Trivial Thinking. Cleaning up your desk because you have buried an important document and need to submit it immediately is Necessity Thinking.

The trick is to always stay in the *Proactive* quadrant (*Important but not urgent*), although it takes discipline. The more time you spend being proactive, the less likely you are to end up in Quadrant 1. You do not want to live in Quadrant 1, the *Necessity* quadrant, as it creates a lot of stress – everything is due tomorrow. This Quadrant is bad for your health! I advise you to spend half of your day on proactive tasks if possible. However, even if you spend 5 min of your day on proactive tasks, then you will have an advantage. In addition, it is important to avoid *Comfort* and *Trivial* tasks. Delegate the *Comfort* and *Trivial* tasks. For example, a senior doctoral student can delegate tasks to junior doctoral and other graduate and undergraduate students because they can perform those tasks. Instead, the senior doctoral student can concentrate on more important tasks without having to perform everything.

Meetings fall under urgent and important tasks. Although meetings consume a major part of your time, it is still a necessity that everyone must meet. However, try to minimize the time of your meetings by being more efficient, having a detailed agenda, and asking participants to stay on task. In general, try to decrease the number of your meetings, if possible, so you have more time to be proactive.

6.2.2   Tips for planning and prioritizing

Below are some tips to improve your planning and prioritizing.

Spend 7 min before you leave to prepare for the next day. If you spend more than that, then you put too much on your list. If you spend more than 7-min thinking about your next day tasks, then you're adding more tasks than you can handle.

Do not over-commit because something new might happen. You want to allocate 50% of your tasks as proactive (Figure 6.1), but you also want to leave time for other tasks that your boss or mentor may ask you to complete, otherwise your "to-do list" will become a mess. Don't over-commit. It's better to have fewer tasks. Then, this frees you to work on proactive tasks.

Have an effective system to organize your tasks and your files. We used to have file folders, but nowadays we can store everything on our computer (folders or emails). I personally use my email (i.e. Outlook) to organize my tasks based on the following folders:

- Inbox – all incoming emails
- Today – all emails that have been read and are associated with tasks I have to do today
- This week – all emails that have been read and are associated with tasks I have to do this week
- Next week – all emails that have been read and are associated with tasks I have to do next week
- Short range – all emails that have been read and are associated with tasks I have to do within the next month
- Long range – all emails that have been read and are associated with tasks I have to do beyond next month
- Pending – all emails which I have addressed but still require input from another person. For example, pending tasks can be a manuscript that I have provided feedback to one of my PhD students, and I am waiting for them to revise and send it back to me.

When I spend my 7 min, I check today's, this week's, and next week's emails/tasks, and I update them. Once a week, I check my short-range and long-range emails/tasks as well as the pending tasks.

In addition, I keep folders on my desktop with the above names (e.g. today), where I keep all the files that I need to complete these tasks. When I am done with a task, I archive the files in directories with the name of the person (i.e. student, collaborator) I worked with on this task.

Eliminate time wasters. The biggest time wasters are as follows:

- Opening junk email. Some people are overly addicted to looking their junk email on a daily basis. It's called junk email for a reason. Leave it and don't waste your time on it! Regarding emailing, see also Vignette 6.1.
- Spending too much time on the phone. First, make calls in blocks of time. Get straight to the point within the first 15 s. It's very frustrating to get a voicemail that only includes a name and a phone number. You can end up playing "phone tag." A good method of avoiding this issue is to leave a detailed message that includes your name, the reason of your call, phone number, and your availability (multiple specific times and dates; e.g. you can call me back on Monday between 3 PM and 3:15 PM).
- Looking for misplaced files. Try to keep your files organized in such a way that fits your needs and requirements.

- Waiting for appointments. Try to minimize the time you waste while waiting for appointments. For example, try to take your laptop, tablet, books, or articles with you when you have a doctor's appointment and read or do your tasks while you are waiting.

Minimize interruptions. You may have several colleagues who love to chat and waste your time when you are busy working.[1] Here are some tips for keeping interruptions for sabotaging your productivity.

- Announce a time. "I have only 10 min."
- Schedule regular meetings if you are frequently interrupted.
- Use the "walk-talk" method. "I am getting ready for my next meeting at the Name Hall. Walk with me and tell me your problem."
- Get to the point assertively.
- Hang a sign on your door.
- Close your door, which is my last resource.

VIGNETTE 6.   Avoid the email trap

Emails are a blessing and a curse. Several people check their emails all the time because they have a notification sound every time they receive an email; that creates distractions. Here are some hints on how to deal with the email trap.

- Check it less often (maybe three times per day). To eliminate the "email addiction," you could take a break every hour and check your emails. Then slowly make these breaks longer. I tend to check them at specific times: first thing in the morning when I start working, after lunch, and close to the end of my working day[2]. *Do not check your emails before you go to bed*, because a frustrating email may affect your sleep.
- Act rather than just reading and re-reading emails by immediately making notes in your calendar and move them in their respective folders (see above my filling system). For example, if you receive an email from your mentor regarding a conference abstract deadline in 7 months, then move it to your long-range folder.

---

[1] A previous colleague of mine was notorious for interrupting people when they were trying to work. He used to spend 15 min in each faculty office to talk about football games. I knew precisely when this person would pass by, and so, I used to close my office door before he showed up.

[2] My boss knows that I do not constantly check my emails … so she calls me.

- Switch off all notifications to eliminate those distractions. I have switched off all notifications related to emails to eliminate distractions with one exception. I leave the notifications on for a specific cross-platform, instant messaging and voice over IP application, because I use this specifically for my family and close friends.

6.2.3   Delegation

As you move along in your career and gain more and more responsibilities you will be required to delegate. Remember that we mentioned above that the Trivial and the Comfort quadrants are "ripe" for delegation. As you move along in your career and gain more and more responsibilities, you will be required to delegate. However, the question is how to delegate. Here is how I organize my delegated tasks.

I have an Excel spreadsheet that includes all tasks that I need to delegate and the personnel who would be able to perform them, what the task requires, and what information they need to be given to be able to complete it. At my end-of-semester individual meetings with my staff and research team, I discuss the tasks that the individual likes and those they detest. I then have a good idea of which tasks should be delegated to whom.

Practically, my spreadsheet contains four columns. The first column is called TO DO, and this is where I write down all my tasks. I update this column once a week. The second column is called COULD ANYONE ELSE DO IT. In this column, I place a minus sign if I believe that I have to do the task myself and a plus sign if I feel I can delegate it. The third column is called WHO. Here I write the names of my people who would be able to perform the tasks based on their evaluations. The fourth column is called WHAT DO THEY NEED TO KNOW. In this column, I include information like the deadline, the outcomes required, etc. If they could do it but need more experience in specific aspects of the task, then I plan educational experiences for them in order to improve their capabilities. This is especially true for frequently occurring tasks.

Delegation is difficult, especially earlier in your career. You would really want to do everything by yourself because you are afraid that other people will make mistakes. However, at that time, remember how many mistakes you made and keep making. You have to live with mistakes and errors because everybody makes them. In order to minimize mistakes and errors caused by delegation, make a strong effort to hire and recruit well. In addition, if you can find people that you work well with, they are diligent and meticulous, and make every effort to maintain them in your staff and your life. You will eventually be as good as the people with which you surround yourself.

6.2.3.1 Recruiting and hiring

To be able to delegate, you need to have capable individuals around in order to be able to assign tasks with minimal fear. However, in general, it is fundamental in order to be successful in any job to be able to recruit and hire well. There are numerous publications from the business world on this topic. Here, I would like to present few personal hints to better accomplish these two tasks.

Recruiting is all about marketing yourself and your environment and enhancing your visibility. To accomplish this, I recommend the following:

- Be present at meetings and walk through as many posters as possible, introducing yourself to students and other presenters. Hand over your business card and the work you present at the meeting in a form of a handout.
- Pave your way with publications.
- Have effective online resources (i.e. website, social media).
- Publish an annual newsletter of your laboratory and your research environment.

Hiring requires diligent work at all levels. You need to interview the candidate, the references of the candidate, and in general, try to learn as much as possible about the candidate. Personally, I also seek the opinions of my other team members. If I am hiring a new faculty member, I seek feedback from every person in my department. My interviews are always intense, and I ask many questions while I keep notes. Below I have provided two lists with possible questions that I use for my interviews. The first is a list of questions that I use for candidates of academic positions (i.e. professors at all levels). The second is a longer list of questions that I use for candidates of graduate assistantships/fellowships and staff positions.

List 1. Questions that I use for candidates of academic positions (i.e. professors at all levels)

1. Why are you interested in this job?
2. How would you describe your teaching philosophy?
3. Do you have any experience in teaching students of non-traditional age? Teaching students from a diversity of social or ethnic backgrounds? Teaching graduate students?
4. How would you go about promoting active learning and a high level of engagement among your students?
5. What is the most interesting book you've read in the past 6 months?

6. Have you done anything that provides evidence of support for inter-disciplinary studies or for academic disciplines outside of your own field?
7. If there were one book that all freshmen in college were required to read, what should it be?
8. What makes you unique as an individual?
9. What part of academic life gives you the most pleasure?
10. What part of academic life annoys you the most, exasperates you, or is a pet peeve?
11. What do you regard as the biggest challenge facing college and university professors today?
12. What is your most significant accomplishment in your present position?
13. What would you regard as the proper balance between scholarship and teaching for a faculty member?
14. What is your greatest strength as a faculty member?
15. If I were to speak to those who know you best, what would they describe as your greatest weakness?
16. What achievements would you like to look back on after your first year as a faculty member here?
17. Describe a mistake that you made in your professional life.
18. Describe a problem that you have solved in your professional life.
19. What do people who don't like you say about you?
20. What are some examples of your creativity and innovation as a teacher?
21. What is your favorite word in the English language? Why?
22. If you could converse with any particular leader or historical figure, who would it be? Why?
23. What three sources do you use most to gain information about recent trends in your field?
24. (Give each candidate a list of the essential job-related functions of the position.) Let's go through this list, and I'd like you to tell me how you would accomplish each of these tasks.
25. If you could develop your knowledge or skills in any one area, what would it be?
26. What do you regard to be the single most important asset for a faculty member in higher education today?

List 2. Questions that I use for candidates of graduate assistantships/fellowships and staff positions

1. Describe a major change that occurred in a job that you held. How did you adapt to this change? Tell us about a situation in which you had to adjust to changes over which you had no control. How did you handle it?

2. Tell us about a time that you had to adapt to a difficult situation.

3. What do you do when priorities change quickly? Give one example of when this happened.

4. Describe a project or idea that was implemented primarily because of your efforts. What was your role? What was the outcome?

5. Describe a time when you made a suggestion to improve the work in your previous work environment.

6. Give an example of an important goal that you set in the past. Tell me about your success in reaching it. Give two examples of things you've done in previous jobs that demonstrate your willingness to work hard.

7. How many hours a day do you put into your work? What were your study patterns at school?

8. Tell us about a time when you had to go above and beyond the call of duty in order to get a job done. Tell us about a time when a job had to be completed and you were able to focus your attention and efforts to get it done.

9. Tell us about a time when you were particularly effective at prioritizing tasks and completing a project on schedule.

10. Tell us about the last time that you undertook a project that demanded a lot of initiative. Tell us how you keep your job knowledge current with the ongoing changes in your area of study.

11. There are times when we work without close supervision or support to get the job done. Tell us about a time when you found yourself in such a situation and how things turned out.

12. What impact did you have in your last job?

13. What is the most competitive work situation you have experienced? How did you handle it? What was the result?

14. What is the riskiest decision you have made? What was the situation? What happened?

15. What kinds of challenges did you face on your last job? Give an example of how you handled them. What projects have you started on your own recently? What prompted you to get started?

16. What sorts of things have you done to become better qualified for your career? What was the best idea that you came up with in your career? How did you apply it? When you disagree with your manager, what do you do? Give an example.

17. When you have a lot of work to do, how do you get it all done? Give an example?

18. Describe the project or situation which best demonstrates your analytical abilities. What was your role?

19. Developing and using a detailed procedure is often very important in a job. Tell about a time when you needed to develop and use a detailed procedure to successfully complete a project.

20. Give me a specific example of a time when you used good judgment and logic in solving a problem. Give me an example of when you took a risk to achieve a goal. What was the outcome?

21. How did you go about making the changes (step by step)? Answer in depth or detail such as "What were you thinking at that point?" or "Tell me more about meeting with that person" or "Lead me through your decision process."

22. Tell us about a job or setting where great attention to detail was required to complete a task. How did you handle that situation?

23. Tell us about a time when you had to analyze information and make a recommendation. What kind of thought process did you go through? What was your reasoning behind your decision?

24. Have you ever worked in a situation where the rules and guidelines were not clear? Tell me about it. How did you feel about it? How did you react?

25. Some people consider themselves to be "big picture people" and others are "detail oriented." Which are you? Give an example of a time when you displayed this.

26. Tell us me about a situation when it was important for you to pay attention to details. How did you handle it?

27. Tell us me about a time when you demonstrated too much initiative?

28. Describe a situation in which you were able to effectively "read" another person and guide your actions by your understanding of their individual needs or values.

29. Describe a situation when you were able to strengthen a relationship by communicating effectively. What made your communication effective?

30. Describe a situation where you felt you had not communicated well. How did you correct the situation? Describe a time when you were able to effectively communicate a difficult or unpleasant idea to a superior.

31. Describe the most significant written document, report or presentation that you have completed. Give me an example of a time when you were able to successfully communicate with another person, even when that individual may not have personally liked you, or vice versa.

32. How do you go about explaining a complex technical problem to a person who does not understand technical jargon? What approach do you take in communicating with people?

33. What kinds of communication situations cause you difficulty? Give an example.

34. Tell us about a recent successful experience in making a speech or presentation. How did you prepare? What obstacles did you face? How did you handle them?

35. Tell us about a time when you and your current/previous supervisor disagreed but you still found a way to get your point across.
36. Tell us about a time when you were particularly effective in a talk you gave or a seminar you taught. Tell us about an experience in which you had to speak up in order to be sure that other people knew what you thought or felt.
37. What are the most challenging documents you have written? What kinds of proposals have you written? What kinds of writing have you done? How do you prepare written communications?
38. Describe a time when you took personal accountability for a conflict and initiated contact with the individual(s) involved to explain your actions.
39. Discuss an important decision you have made regarding a task or project at work. What factors influenced your decision?
40. Everyone has made some poor decisions or has done something that just did not turn out right. Has this happened to you? What happened?
41. Describe a situation where you had the option to leave the details to others or you could take care of them yourself.
42. Do you prefer to work with the "big picture" or the "details" of a situation? Give me an example of an experience that illustrates your preference.
43. Have the jobs you held in the past required little attention, moderate attention, or a great deal of attention to detail? Give me an example of a situation that illustrates this requirement.
44. Have you ever had a situation where you had a number of alternatives to choose from? How did you go about choosing one?
45. How did you assemble the information?
46. How did you review the information? What process did you follow to reach a conclusion? What alternatives did you develop?
47. How have you adjusted your style when it was not meeting the objectives and/or people were not responding correctly?
48. What do you do when you are faced with an obstacle to an important project? Give an example. When you have difficulty persuading someone to your point of view, what do you do? Give an example.
49. How did you keep track of delegated assignments?
50. How do you evaluate the productivity/effectiveness of your subordinates? How do you get data for performance reviews?
51. Give me an example of when you had to go above and beyond the call of duty in order to get a job done.
52. Give me examples of projects/tasks you started on your own.
53. Give some instances in which you anticipated problems and were able to influence a new direction.

54. Describe a recent unpopular decision you made and what the result was.
55. Tell us about the most difficult or frustrating individual that you've ever had to work with, and how you managed to work with them.
56. What have you done in the past to contribute towards a teamwork environment?
57. Can you think of a situation where innovation was required at work? What did you do in this situation?
58. Describe a time when you came up with a creative solution/idea/project/report to a problem in your past work.
59. Describe a time when you were asked to keep information confidential.
60. Give examples of how you have acted with integrity in your job/work relationship.
61. If you can, tell about a time when your trustworthiness was challenged. How did you react/respond? On occasion we are confronted by dishonesty in the workplace. Tell about such an occurrence and how you handled it.
62. Tell us about a specific time when you had to handle a tough problem which challenged fairness or ethnical issues.
63. Trust requires personal accountability. Can you tell about a time when you chose to trust someone? What was the outcome?
64. Have you ever met resistance when implementing a new idea or policy to a work group? How did you deal with it? What happened?
65. When is the last time you had to introduce a new idea or procedure to people on the job? How did you do it?
66. Give an example of your ability to build motivation in your co-workers, classmates, and even if on a volunteer committee.
67. Have you ever had difficulty getting others to accept your ideas? What was your approach? Did it work?
68. Have you ever been a member of a group where two of the members did not work well together? What did you do to get them to do so?
69. Give an example of a time when you made a mistake because you did not listen well to what someone had to say.
70. How often do you have to rely on information you have gathered from others when talking to them? What kinds of problems have you had? What happened?
71. What do you do to show people that you are listing to them?
72. Have you ever had a subordinate whose work was always marginal? How did you deal with that person? What happened?
73. How do you deal with people whose work exceeds your expectations?
74. Describe a situation when you were able to have a positive influence on the actions of others. Give an example of a time when you went above and beyond the call of duty.

75. Tell us about an important goal that you set in the past. Were you successful? Why?
76. Describe the most challenging negotiation in which you were involved. What did you do? What were the results for you? What were the results for the other party?
77. Have you ever been in a situation where you had to bargain with someone? How did you feel about this? What did you do? Give an example.
78. Describe a time when you had to make a difficult choice between your personal and professional life. Give me an example of a project that best describes your organizational skills.
79. How do you decide what gets top priority when scheduling your time?
80. What do you do when your schedule is suddenly interrupted? Give an example.
81. Give an example of a time when you helped a staff member accept change and make the necessary adjustments to move forward. What were the change/transition skills that you used?
82. How do you handle performance reviews? Tell me about a difficult one.
83. Tell us about a time when you had to take disciplinary action with someone you supervised.
84. Tell us about a time when you had to tell a staff member that you were dissatisfied with his or her work.
85. When do you give positive feedback to people? Tell me about the last time you did. Give an example of how you handle the need for constructive criticism with a subordinate or peer.
86. Give an example of a situation where others were intense but you were able to maintain your composure.
87. It is important to maintain a positive attitude at work when you have other things on your mind. Give a specific example of when you were able to do that.
88. Describe how you develop a project team's goals and project plan?
89. How do you schedule your time? Set priorities? How do you handle multi-tasking?
90. What do you do when your time schedule or project plan is upset by unforeseen circumstances? Give an example.
91. What have you done in order to be effective with your organization and planning?
92. How do you prepare for a presentation to a group of technical experts in your field? How would you describe your presentation style?
93. Tell us about the most effective presentation you have made. What was the topic? What made it difficult? How did you handle it?

94. What kinds of oral presentations have you made? How did you prepare for them? What challenges did you have?

95. Describe the most difficult working relationship you've had with an individual. What specific actions did you take to improve the relationship? What was the outcome?

96. Give me an example of a situation where you had difficulties with a team member. What, if anything, did you do to resolve the difficulties?

97. Have you ever been caught unaware by a problem or obstacles that you had not foreseen? What happened?

98. Have you ever been in a situation where you had to settle an argument between two friends (or people you knew)? What did you do? What was the result?

99. Have you ever had to settle conflict between two people on the job? What was the situation and what did you do?

100. Tell us about a time when you had to help two peers settle a dispute. How did you go about identifying the issues? What did you do? What was the result?

101. Tell us about a time when you organized or planned an event that was very successful.

102. Can you recall a time when you were less than pleased with your performance?

103. Give me an example of an important goal that you had set in the past and tell me about your success in reaching it.

104. If there were one area you've always wanted to improve upon, what would that be? In what ways are you trying to improve yourself?

105. Have you ever been overloaded with work? How do you keep track of work so that it gets done on time?

106. How do you manage your time? How do you schedule your time?

107. When given an important assignment, how do you approach it?

108. Describe a situation when you had to exercise a significant amount of self-control.

109. Give me an example of a time in which you had to be relatively quick in coming to a decision.

110. Give me an example of when you were able to meet the personal and professional demands in your life yet still maintained a healthy balance.

111. How did you react when faced with constant time pressure? Give an example.

112. What is the most stressful situation you have faced? How did you deal with it?

113. Describe a situation in which you had to arrive at a compromise or help others to compromise. What was your role? What steps did you take? What was the end result?

114. Describe a team experience you found disappointing. What would you have done to prevent this?
115. Describe a team experience you found rewarding.
116. Describe the types of teams with which you've been involved. What were your roles?
117. Have you ever been in a position where you had to lead a group of peers? How did you handle it?
118. Tell us about setbacks you have faced. How did you deal with them?
119. What has been your major work related disappointment? What happened and what did you do?

6.3   Laboratory management

In order to become a successful scientist, it is very important to know how to effectively manage your laboratory. The following is a list of different practices I follow based on the overwhelming amount of advice I have received over the years from scientists much more experienced than me. I specifically want to acknowledge two individuals that have influenced me significantly in this area, my PhD mentor Dr. Barry Bates and Dr. Walter Herzog of the University of Calgary.

6.3.1   Be an effective laboratory head and manager

To be an effective laboratory head and manager, you need to be a leader. I personally feel that this only happens when you lead by example. You need to match their effort, and you need to set goals that you will follow through with them. In this fashion, you will eventually inspire your people to follow you. However, on a daily basis, a manager's effectiveness comes down to the following tasks:

- Prioritize responsibilities. This is accomplished by
  - Setting goals.
  - Communicating.
  - Motivating.
  - Encouraging teamwork.
  - Delegating.
  - Solving problems that may arise.
- Form positive work habits. This is accomplished by
  - Training your team.
  - Being open to change.
  - Being a team member.
  - Providing recognition.
  - Showing concern.

- Take charge when needed. This is accomplished by
  - Being available and visible.
  - Being confident.
  - Avoid making sudden changes.
  - Listening.
  - Always matching and even surpassing their effort.
- Establish credibility and gain commitment. This is accomplished by
  - Being fair and consistent.
  - Involving your team in decision making.
  - Having a positive attitude.
  - Being proactive.
  - Accepting responsibilities for mistakes.
  - Being respectful.
  - Enjoying your job.
  - Recognizing excellence and confronting and correcting poor performance.
- Manage people's perceptions. For example, your body language is very important, how you sit, how you walk, how you dress, etc. In terms of how you dress, I like to wear dark colors, which demonstrate more power. I also use a black uniform for my entire staff. Initially we wore lab coats but we also wanted to differentiate ourselves from the medical center. Therefore, we decided on a lab polo shirt that was black. We combine this polo shirt with black pants as our uniform to reflect strength.

6.3.2   My personal practices

I have a list of activities that I have followed ever since I started my academic career in order to be an effective manager and head.

6.3.2.1   Weekly reports

I learned about weekly reports from my PhD mentor. We used to type them and then pin them on a cork board Monday morning outside his door. I adopted this practice as soon as I started working as a faculty member. Even now as an administrator, I require my staff to submit weekly reports, which I expect in my inbox by 8 AM on Monday morning. Many of my colleagues have adopted this practice of mine and have mentioned to me on numerous occasions how this has helped them in their laboratory management.

The weekly reports are divided in three areas; tasks that were accomplished last week, tasks that are planned for the following week, and outstanding tasks. Under outstanding tasks, someone could include pending tasks (i.e. a submitted paper), items that are of less priority because they belong to long-range planning, etc. I also allow individualization of the weekly reports as some people would like to add more categories or additional details. In Vignette 6.2, I have included an exemplary weekly report from a previous doctoral student of mine.

VIGNETTE 6.2   Exemplary weekly report

NAME
Weekly report: DATE
Last week (tasks accomplished): DATES
Projects:

Project 1. Dissertation:

Task 1: Review stats from second Part B manuscript given advice on covariates from our biostatistician.

Accomplished: She believes that the problems I'm experiencing are because there are too many terms in the model given that I have a small sample size.

Task 2: Meet with my assigned undergraduate student regarding work tasks.

Accomplished: Done. She is working on categorizing the foot contacts using the video data. She met twice with me to make sure we'd classify them the same way, and to discuss some of the things she had already found.

Task 3: Arrange time to meet with Dr. Stergiou to discuss requirements for dissertation, for example, number and content of manuscripts.

Accomplished: Done. Met with Dr. Stergiou. I have been working on how best to structure and order the papers in my dissertation based on our discussion, and how to show the progression of my original model.

Additional Accomplishments: I am trying to work out a good way of determining how to quantify how the variability of the movements of the different segments changes over time to achieve an overall reduction of variability on the uneven ground. I also did some more Part C tracking.

Project 2. Variability and falls:
No work last week.

Project 3. R15:
No work last week.

Papers:

Task 1. Continue revising first Part B manuscript.

Accomplished: I did a small amount on this.

Task 2. Continue bullet pointing second Part B manuscript for feedback.

Accomplished. I didn't do anything on this as I was still trying to work out how best to analyze the data. Having spoken to Dr. Stergiou, I believe that this manuscript might be omitted as I think the others that I am planning will be more profitable, answer more targeted questions, and add more to my model.

Task 3. Aim to complete rough draft of first Part A manuscript.

Accomplished. I completed a very rough draft of the manuscript minus abstract and conclusion paragraph. It still needs a lot of work before anyone sees it.

Grants:

No work last week.

Miscellaneous:

Accomplished: I attended the XXXXXXX Symposium at XXXXXX University. It was extremely interesting and relevant to my dissertation work.

This week (tasks planned): DATES
Projects:

Project 1. Dissertation:

Task 1. Meet with my assigned undergraduate student regarding work tasks.

Task 2. Track more Part C data.

Task 3. Work out if Principal Component Analysis is appropriate. If so, write code for it and run through data from a couple of participants.

Project 2. Variability and falls:
No work is planned.

Project 3. R15:

Task 1. Compile paperwork for VA Institutional Review Board completion report.

Papers:

Task 1. Continue revising first Part B manuscript when time is available.

Task 2. Work on completing a less rough discussion and conclusion for first Part A manuscript.

Task 3. Start on methods section for second Part A manuscript.

Grants:

No work is planned.

Miscellaneous:

Attend faculty interview (Monday).

Outstanding Items

Papers:

Submitted:

None at this time.

In progress:

Dissertation Part B.

Planned:

R15 paper on balance.

Grants:

Currently funded:

R15

Grant for dissertation project.

Submitted:

None at this time.

Planned:

None at this time.

Projects:

Project 1. Dissertation

Data collection – 26/26 complete, +1 incomplete

Data tracking – 2.5/30 complete entirely; 11/11 complete for Part A; 11/63 trials complete for Part C1

Project 2. Vibration project

Data collection completed

Session 1: 18/30 control participants collected, 20/30 amputee participants collected

Session 2: 18/30 control participants collected, 17/30 amputee participants collected (4 amputee/1 control participants did overground trials only)

6.3.2.2   Individual meetings

I utilize individual meetings every week. These are meeting with my staff and the members of my research team. They are usually short, around 15 min, and based on the weekly reports. Their main goal is to address items of immediate concern and to answer any immediate questions.

6.3.2.3   Team meetings

I meet with my research team (undergraduate and graduate students, research associates, etc.) every other week. This is called a team meeting and lasts 60 min. One of the students is responsible to prepare the agenda and to type the minutes as we discuss everything. We go over all the projects without discussing findings, mostly just business-related items. We address issues related to data collections, data analysis, informed consents, equipment, recruiting, etc. We also go over all the manuscripts and grants we have active, pending, or in progress. Lastly, we discuss submission of abstracts and presentations in conferences.

6.3.2.4   Data meetings

The in-between weeks when I don't have team meetings, I organize data meetings that last 60–90 min. During these meetings, my research team discusses results from the different projects we have in progress, ideas, grant submissions, etc. The format is slide-based presentations where exchange of ideas and feedback is emphasized. Our team members get 15–30 min for presentation and discussion. We usually have three to four projects per meeting.

6.3.2.5   Journal clubs

For the team and data meetings, I usually target Mondays. However, for the Journal Club I target Fridays or another day towards the end of the week. It lasts 60 min. My entire research team participates, and the goal is to discuss three to four scientific papers that we have read. I require from the participants to have critically analyzed the papers. I don't expect anyone to present the papers as we move directly into its critique. Questions such as what you like and don't like in this paper are usually the first posed. I emphasize critical thinking and discussion. Many times, I give assignments such as digging deeper in the literature with respect to a specific topic. I usually identify the scientific papers that we are going to read. However, I also encourage team members to step forward to identify papers that they would like everyone to read.

For journal clubs, many times I ask my team to meet outside the University; a coffee shop, a diner, even a pub. The goal is to promote a sense of being away from a classroom and to encourage participants to express opinions more freely. The majority of my doctoral students and research associates consider our journal clubs the most important educational experience of their time with me. One of them placed a coffee mug from the place where we used to meet on the first page of his dissertation. Another mentioned it in her acknowledgments. Therefore, I strongly encourage having journal clubs and pay particular attention in the selection of the papers to be discussed.

6.3.2.6   The laboratory notebook

As it should be for every laboratory, all the members of my research team are required to keep a laboratory notebook. This serves as their record of the research they perform and where you can find their logical trees. In their laboratory notebook, they document their hypotheses, experiments, data analysis, and data interpretation. It is also their moral responsibility as researchers in terms of ethical recording of data, which is a major concern of the scientific community. In Figure 6.2, you can see few pages from the laboratory notebooks of two great scientists, Alexander Graham Bell and Leonardo da Vinci.

A laboratory notebook has several roles. It is a complete record of procedures, data, and thoughts to pass on to other researchers. It is an explanation of why experiments were initiated, how they were performed, and the results. It is a legal document to prove patents and defend your data against accusations of fraud. Lastly, it is the scientific legacy of the laboratory.

Here is an interesting historical example of the importance of keeping a good laboratory notebook. Pierre Charles Le Monnier, a French astronomer, obtains no credit for discovery of planet Uranus, even though he observed Uranus 12 times between 1750 and 1769, including 6 times in 8 days in 1769, without realizing it wasn't a star. He wrote all his measurements on scraps of paper, including a paper bag that had once contained hair powder. Discovery of Uranus as a planet is awarded to British William Herschel, who observed Uranus on March 13, 1781 (Linton, 2004). There are many more interesting cases in the history of science regarding notebooks like the Mycogen Plant Science, Inc. v. Monsanto Co. lawsuit; the excellent record of the First Transistor Amplifier in the AT&T Bell Labs by Walter H. Brattain in December 24, 1947 (resulted in him getting a Nobel Prize); and more recently, in 2011, the Judy Mikovits case who was a biochemist that was arrested and jailed on a felony charge of possessing stolen property from a research institute that fired her in September. The property at issue consisted of her laboratory notebooks and related data (Cohen, 2011).

There are various types of laboratory notebooks, a Bound/Stitched Notebook, a Loose Leaf/Three Ring Binder Notebook, and/or an Electronic Notebook. I personally prefer a Bound/Stitched Notebook where pages are difficult to be removed and always available to make notes. I also prefer notebooks that are large, at least 8.5×11, so it is easier

(a)

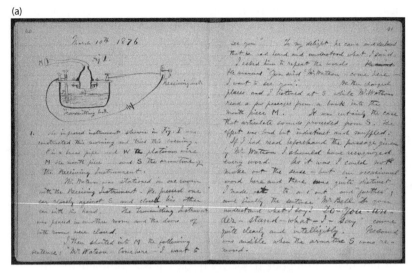

(b)

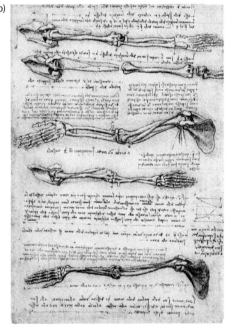

Figure 6.2 Pages from the laboratory notebooks of two great scientists: (a) Alexander Graham Bell – pages 40–41 of Alexander Graham Bell Family Papers in the Library of Congress' Manuscript Division, Public Domain, https://commons.wikimedia.org/w/index.php?curid=7785180; (b) Leonardo da Vinci – his notebook regarding the study of the arm, Public Domain, https://commons.wikimedia.org/w/index.php?curid=59576.

to attach different materials. I like them to be white gridded made by acid-free paper which can last for almost 30 years (as patents take time to be issued and your notebook should last 23 years after patent issue).

The notebook should have your name and year in the inside cover or cover page as well as a general project name, and the lab mailing address. Then, it should include a Table of Contents (that is updated as you write the rest of the notebook) and the experimental entries along with their logical trees. The experimental entries should be organized as follows:

- Date
- Title
- Hypothesis or Goal: Brief statement of purpose
- Background: Logical tree
- How: Protocols, calculations, equipment
- Observations:
  - All that happens (planned or unplanned – you never know what may be important)
  - Raw experimental data
  - Taped-in information or reference to data location
- Data analysis:
  - Processing of raw data, graphs, interpretations statistical methods used
- Ideas for future experiments – better controls, etc.
- Additional materials
  - Emails
  - Notes of discussions and conversations
  - Photographs
  - Printed graphs

Every page of the notebook should have a number which will make the construction of the Table of Contents much easier. In addition, every entry should be dated and signed. All data go in to the notebook, even "bad" data points or "outliers." Any failed experiments or contradictory experiments should be included. No pages should come out of the notebook or be skipped. Unused parts of a page should be crossed out. Data should never be removed. Mistakes should be corrected and not removed. Correction of mistakes could be done by crossing them with a single line. In addition, all mistakes should be signed and dated.

All entries in the notebook should be made using a ballpoint pen with permanent black or blue ink. Pencils, erasures, or white-outs should never be used. Writing should be legible and clear. It should be detailed so someone else in your discipline could understand the procedures and repeat them. Drawings and flow charts could be included to improve clarity and all abbreviations should be defined.

Work should be recorded in the notebook as it is performed and as soon as possible. The best of course is today and at the latest it should be recorded the next day. A weekly checkup should be performed to make sure that all experimental conditions are provided, all results have been recorded, all summaries are written, future directions are stated, the Table of Contents has been updated, and everything (photos, etc.) is attached securely.

6.3.3   Daily rituals of the greats – how the greats organized their days

In a recent book, Currey (2013) details the sleep, work, and recreational habits of several famous historical figures during certain periods of their lives. All of these people were extremely successful, but they followed very different schedules. The most common characteristic of all but one of these great figures is that they did not actually spend an intense amount of time on their work. They slept an average of 7 h, socialized and exercised. This may have led them to be more focused and efficient in their work. All these great men were normal people, and the take home message is that you don't have to perform impossible feats to be like them.

6.3.3.1   The musicians

Ludwig van Beethoven (1770–1827, German; evidence dated 1822–1827). Beethoven was a balanced person. He slept for 8 h (from 10 PM to 6 AM) and after a short 30-min breakfast, he worked for another 8 h. In the afternoon, he walked for 2 h with manuscript paper and a pencil in his pocket to write down ideas that came to him, upon which he would find a tree to support his paper. He had several hours of leisure time in the evening, during which he would read a newspaper at a local tavern, drink beer, and smoke a pipe.

Wolfgang Amadeus Mozart (1756–1791, Austrian; evidence dated 1781). Mozart, on the other hand, used to sleep only 5 h per night. He spent an hour dressing as he was a very social man and into fashion. In the morning he then spent 2 h composing, followed by 4 h of music lessons as he needed the money from teaching music. He had a long lunch (almost 4 h) during which he socialized. In the early evenings, he composed or performed for 4 h, and then, at this time, spent a couple of hours courting Constanze (he loved courting). He often then used to compose until 1 o'clock in the morning and be back up again at 6 AM. So, to sum it up, he spent 8 h composing but with long interruptions, 4 h teaching, 5 h sleeping, and the rest of his time having fun. Thus, he practically worked 12 h which is much more than Beethoven and slept less in order to socialize.

6.3.3.2 The writers

Honoré de Balzac (1799–1850, French; historical period unidentified). Balzac, the famous French writer, was a very interesting man regarding the organization of his day. He spent over 13 h a day writing, fueled by as many as 50 cups of black coffee per day! He chose to go to sleep from 6 PM then wake at 1 AM to start writing. With a nap from 8 AM until 9:30 AM, he ended up with 8.5 h of sleep each day. He exercised for half an hour and received visitors for only an hour and a half. He sacrificed his social life for work.

Charles Dickens (1812–1870, English; evidence dated 1851–1860). Dickens was continuously working against deadlines because he had his own Victorian periodical. This was a weekly literary magazine published between 1859 and 1895 throughout the United Kingdom. It hosted the serialization of many prominent novels, including Dickens' own A Tale of Two Cities.[3] Despite this, he slept for 7 h (midnight to 7 AM), exercised for 3 h vigorously walking through the streets of London, and spent most of the rest of his time with his family, only working for 5 h.

6.3.3.3 The scientists

Sigmund Freud (1856–1939, Austrian; evidence dated 1910). Freud used to sleep for only 6 h (from 1 AM to 7 AM) and work for 12.5 h. Most of his work time was devoted to seeing patients and his writing for scientific journals was mostly at night between 10:30 PM and 1 AM. After a break and lunch, in the afternoon he would also exercise, which involved walking around Vienna at high speed. An hour and a half in the evening was spent eating supper and walking with his wife or daughter. He sacrificed his family time for his patients and his work.

Charles Darwin (1809–1882, English; evidence dated 1842–1859). Darwin slept 7 h (midnight to 7 AM), then woke up, went for a walk, and ate breakfast before starting work at about 8 AM. He worked for a total of 10 h, but his work pattern was erratic, interspersed with walking, reading, writing letters, and spending time with his wife, Emma. At night he would lie awake in bed solving problems. He exercised by having three 30-min walks around the day.

Nikola Tesla (1856–1943, Serbian-American; evidence dated 1900–1922). Tesla worked every day from 9 AM until 6 PM or later. He had dinner at 8:10 PM at Delmonico's restaurant and later the Waldorf-Astoria Hotel. The meal was required to be ready at 8 PM. He usually dined alone. On some occasions, he would eat with a group due to certain social obligations. Tesla would then work till 3 AM, and he would never sleep more

---

[3] In those times, there were no televisions. Dickens wrote a series for a magazine that was extremely famous. It was shipped to America, and each installment of his series was so hotly anticipated that people would shout to the workers on the incoming boats to find out what happened next in the story.

than 2h per night. However, he did admit to taking short power naps from time to time. Tesla also walked between 8 and 10 miles per day. The information regarding Tesla was acquired from O'Neill (1944).

Benjamin Franklin (1706–1790, American; evidence dated 1771). Franklin was both a scientist and a politician. He used to get 7h of sleep per night (from 10 PM to 5 AM) and worked an 8-h day. He did not exercise, but had a significant amount of rest, social time, reflection, and prayer time. He lived by 13 virtues (Vignette 6.2), which he developed at the age of 20 and continued to practice in some form for the rest of his life. Several of them apply directly to time management and organization. Interestingly, his first thought of a morning was "What good shall I do today?" Before going to bed he evaluated; "What good have I done today?"

VIGNETTE 6.3   Benjamin Franklin's 13 virtues

As listed in his autobiography (Franklin, 1996)

1. Temperance. Eat not to dullness; drink not to elevation.
2. Silence. Speak not but what may benefit others or yourself; avoid trifling conversation.
3. Order. Let all your things have their places; let each part of your business have its time.
4. Resolution. Resolve to perform what you ought; perform without fail what you resolve.
5. Frugality. Make no expense but do good to others or yourself; i.e. waste nothing.
6. Industry. Lose no time; be always employed in something useful; cut off all unnecessary actions.
7. Sincerity. Use no hurtful deceit; think innocently and justly; and, if you speak, speak accordingly.
8. Justice. Wrong none by doing injuries, or omitting the benefits that are your duty.
9. Moderation. Avoid extremes; forbear resenting injuries so much as you think they deserve.
10. Cleanliness. Tolerate no uncleanliness in body, clothes, or habitation.
11. Tranquility. Be not disturbed at trifles, or at accidents common or unavoidable.
12. Chastity. Rarely use venery but for health or offspring, never to dullness, weakness, or the injury of your own or another's peace or reputation.
13. Humility. Imitate Jesus and Socrates.

6.3.4 Examples of amazing modern-day scientists in terms of time management and organization

6.3.4.1 Alfredo Quiñones-Hinojosa

Alfredo Quiñones-Hinojosa is a neurosurgeon, author, and researcher. Currently, he is the William J. and Charles H. Mayo Professor and Chair of Neurologic Surgery and runs a basic science research lab at the Mayo Clinic in Jacksonville, Florida. In 2011, Ledford highlighted his work schedule in an article in *Nature* (Ledford, 2011). The title of the article was the 24/7 lab and presented a scientist with a very intense work ethic. Dr. Quiñones-Hinojosa had an unbelievable talent and drive that kept motivating him through his path from being a 19-year-old immigrant from Mexico knowing no English and laboring on fruit farms in California to a prominent neurosurgeon at a leading research institution.[4] The article states that he sleeps 4 h per day and works practically the rest. His laboratory never stops producing, but at the same time, everybody is motivated to work with him. How can he achieve such a feat? Below I have listed some thoughts.

Passion. Dr. Quiñones has a clear philosophy that involves following an extreme regimen to achieve a certain goal. He likens attempting to go "the extra step" to training your brain like an athlete. Why does Dr. Quiñones keep working endless hours every week? *He has a passion for what he is doing*, which drives him to work endless hours to achieve the impossible. He invites patients into the lab to attend his team meetings. That's a great idea. It gives you the real-life perspective to remind you how important the work that you are doing is. It's a great motivation for you and your team. We are fortunate in Biomechanics, as there is a lot of interaction during data collection sessions, through which we often have the privilege of hearing the personal stories of our participants. This is one of the motivating factors that specifically drew me to clinical biomechanics. I would find it hard to motivate myself when working at the molecular level.

Volume. At the time that the article was published, Dr. Quiñones' team held 13 funded grants and had published 113 articles in the previous 6 years. What is the secret to this academic success?

"It's just a matter of volume…The key is we submit a couple of dozen grant applications a year, and we learn from our mistakes." They have published an average of 19 papers/year, which indicates their hard-working spirit and hunger for academic success. You must submit papers and grant applications first to know your mistakes. I always speak to my students about a game I played when I was young, basketball. It is all

---

[4] His story can be read in Quiñones-Hinojosa, Terra Firma – A Journey from Migrant Farm Labor to Neurosurgery. *N. Engl. J. Med.* 357, 529–531 (2007). He is not the only one with such a story.

about the rebounds and the loose balls. They will give you more shots, and the more you shoot, the more you increase your chance of scoring and winning. In addition, if you don't practice shooting the basketball, you will not learn from your mistakes and become better. There is no way around this. For every grant for which you receive funding, the next ten will not be funded. Stay humble and accept the criticism you are given, and do not blame others for your own mistakes.

A good fit. Dr. Quiñones' students love hard work and follow his philosophy. Two of his employees left the lab because they did not want to keep attending the Friday evening lab meetings! At least mine are with beer! You must interact with people in the environment that you think you are interested in joining to gather information about their work ethic and make sure it fits with yours. Based on that information, you can decide if you want to join that lab or not.

Autonomy. Despite the work ethic of his lab, Dr. Quiñones' students still feel that they are free to set their own schedules. I have realized over the years that giving autonomy in terms of scheduling is critical for scientists.

Is this what is needed to achieve success? One of the main reasons that I like Dr. Quiñones' approach is because it follows my philosophy: *you cannot outsmart anyone, but you can outwork everybody.* Of course, this does not mean that all laboratories should work in this fashion to achieve academic success. You may work less than this but more effectively. Dr. Quiñones made multiple sacrifices to his personal life and rarely had time to see his kids. In my opinion, you can find a balance between your family and your job. There are many scientists who have found balance between work and family. However, in all of them, you always observe focused hard work for extended periods of time during the day, excellent time management and organization skills, and certainly a passion for science.

6.3.4.2 Anthony Fauci

Anthony Fauci is an American immunologist who has made substantial contributions to HIV/AIDS research, both as a scientist and as the head of the National Institute of Allergy and Infectious Diseases (NIAID). In 2012, Cohen published an article where the daily life of the Dr. Fauci is presented (Cohen, 2012). As the head of a large National Institutes of Health (NIH) institution, the NIAID, Dr. Fauci is an excellent example of someone who successfully manages to juggle competing tasks at a high level. Through the account of his work day (which starts at 6.30 AM and finishes at 7 PM), we see him in his role as manager, clinician, businessperson, husband, and father. He personally visits patients 3 days a week, despite having his own lab and an important role with the NIH. With all this, he still manages to find time to exercise. How can he perform such a feat? Below I have listed some thoughts.

Proactive. Dr. Fauci dedicates most of his day to proactive content. He finished preparing his talk for a scientific meeting 2 months early. If he can live in the proactive quadrant, anyone else can do it.

Delegate. Dr. Fauci has a good research team that gathers at 5 PM every day to discuss experiments, papers, and revisit their logical tree. He delegates the actual laboratory work and most of the writing to them. However, he is there every step of the way with them conceptually.

Time management. Dr. Fauci has strict rules for email communications to cut down time wasters (*No email longer than one page!*).

Humble. Dr. Fauci stayed 30 min at the end of the day (6:30 PM) to speak with two high-school female students who interviewed him on global ethics.

Many administrators (deans, directors, etc.) stop attending research seminars, teaching, conducting research, and holding reading clubs, which leads to a reduction in academic quality. I know someone that could not teach when he went back to being a professor after being a dean, which led to depression. If you move up in academia, try to maintain your academic obligations alongside your administrative obligations. In addition, try to always stay humble and relate to everyone who works under you.

6.3.5   How I organize my day

Many fellow scientists, students, and others ask me frequently how I organize my work day. Below I have listed this information as it may be of importance to the reader of this book:

5 AM: I get up early and then I meditate/pray for about an hour.

6 AM: Communicate with my family and friends overseas to be able to speak with them despite the 8-h time difference.

6:30 AM: I exercise for an hour mostly lifting weights and performing calisthenics.

7:30 AM: Quick breakfast and then immediately over to my office or 2 h of work in complete silence and then over to my office.

1 PM: Short break for lunch and a short half an hour walk.

5:30 PM: Return home and have dinner.

6:30 PM: Leisure with friends and family for 1–2 h.

8:30 PM: Leisure reading theology, history, or general literature from books identified by my good-friend and amazing Greek writer Mr. Isidoros Zourgos.

10:00 PM: Good night!

Note 1: I always work on Saturdays following closely the above calendar. However, I usually work from my home office.

Note 2: I never work on Sundays. I attend Liturgy at an Orthodox Church in Omaha in the morning and spend the rest of my day on recreational activities (mostly reading my favorite books or watching an educational show on TV).

References

Cohen, J. (2011). Dispute over Lab Notebooks lands researcher in jail. *Science*, 334(6060), 1189–1190.

Cohen, J. (2012). The view from the top of the HIV/AIDS world. *Science*, 337(6091), 152–153.

Currey, M. (2013). *Daily Rituals: How Artists Work*. New York: Knopf Publishers.

Franklin, B. (1996). *The Autobiography of Benjamin Franklin*. New York: Dover Thrift Editions.

Ledford, H. (2011). Working weekends. Leaving at midnight. Friday evening meetings. Does science come out the winner? The 24/7 lab. *Nature*, 477, 20–22.

Linton, C.M. (2004). *From Eudoxus to Einstein: A History of Mathematical Astronomy*. Cambridge: Cambridge University Press.

O'Neill, J.J. (1944). *Prodigal Genius: The Life of Nikola Tesla*. New York: Ives Washburn.

chapter seven

The necessary tasks

I am indebted to my father for living, but to my teacher for living well.

—Alexander the Great: A Greek king and leader (356–323 BC). His teacher was Aristotle.

7.1   Introduction

This chapter discusses a number of important general skills that are needed in order to become a successful scientist and academician. These skills range the spectrum from teaching a class to how to negotiate a deal. You may find some of these skills and my advices to be almost trivial. However, I assure you that at some point in your career you will need every single one of them. In addition, most of the information presented in this chapter applies to employment in the industry and even life in general.

7.2   Working in academia

Getting a job in academia as a tenure-track Assistant Professor or a Lecturer usually occurs after obtaining a PhD or most likely now days a postdoc. In my discipline, Biomechanics, you can still get such a position without a postdoc and in your late 20s or early 30s. This is not the case in other disciplines where competition for academic positions is fierce. Scientists usually complete multiple postdocs and obtain a tenured track position in late 30s or even early 40s.

After you gain such a position, the clock starts in order to obtain tenure which usually occurs in your sixth year. Many young scientists are overstressed regarding the tenure decision, but my advice is to completely ignore it and never think about it. If you do what you love doing, which is science, then you will find it easy to publish your work, obtain grants to perform your work, and teach about what you love working on. Your passion will carry you every minute. By the time you graduate with your PhD, you will have almost 10 years of education and this is certainly enough time to understand if you love science or not. This is fundamental in terms of your success in academia. Being a professor should not only be about teaching or research. It is the combination. It is my opinion that if you only love teaching, you can certainly find a position in a high school, but being at the university, the expectation is that you also perform quality research and contribute to science. At the same time, you teach your graduate and undergraduate students about a subject in which you are an expert, and it is important that you also inspire young minds to be the next generation of scientists and to appreciate what you are doing in the laboratory. It is this excitement about science and research that separates the good teachers from the rest. Furthermore, the skills you have obtained during your graduate education and your postdoc years, will soon be obsolete if you do not use them and keep improving them. Again, this will only happen through research. One of my early role models in my university, Dr. Sheldon Hendricks, who was an extremely successful teacher, mentor, and scientist, used to say, "I can only grow in my teaching through research."

After obtaining tenure (or may even before if this university is not the right environment for you), another decision that you may have to make is when to move to the next level in your career. This level could be combining what you are already doing with administrative duties or going to an environment that offers you better facilities and collaborations you did not have before. Such a move could allow you more personal growth and greater capabilities. In addition, moving to another environment could also occur for personal reasons such as getting closer to family members. The general wisdom states that major moves could occur after 10 years in a certain location/position. In general, it is not advised to move a lot since that gives the impression of one that is not able to settle in one place. Moving to a new position should be well calculated. The grass is not always greener on the other side of the fence. You should consider all factors (i.e. family, start-up funds, expectations, personal growth). My advice is to get to know your future environment as much as possible. This is similar to finding a mentor and a laboratory to pursue graduate work (see chapter five). Speak with everybody and anybody from your new environment, visit several times, and explore how well you will be able to fit in to your new academic home.

7.2.1 Start-up funds

For all the above, a very important factor that you need to consider is the start-up funds. Start-up funds refer to the funds provided by the university that will allow the newly hired faculty member to start effectively the new position. These funds are usually part of the negotiations that will take place beforehand. A frequent question is: what should compose the start-up funds, or, in a more general fashion, what should I ask for?

7.2.1.1 Salary
What you will ask and get as your first salary is very important since it will dictate future salary increases. This is because future salary increases

are usually given as a percentage of your current salary, regardless if such increases are part of a faculty union negotiation (many universities are unionized) or part of a merit increase that is based on your productivity. A larger salary can also be achieved if you can be hired at a higher position (e.g. associate, full professor). However, this is extremely difficult for a young faculty member just after a postdoc; it could be desirable though if you have already grown in your career.

You should also do your research regarding the salary you will seek. If you are applying to a U.S. state-based university, then their salaries are required to be posted online. This will allow you to negotiate within specific limits instead of asking for an unattainable amount. If you are applying to a private university, you can also explore neighboring state universities. In addition, you should examine carefully the living cost as it will affect your net income. Moreover, make sure you negotiate summer opportunities, as most academic contracts will not involve summer payment.

7.2.1.2 Workload

A critical part of the initial negotiations is also the workload that will be given to you. For example, if you are asked to teach 50% or more, you may not have sufficient time to perform your research, as much of your time will be spend in preparing for your classes, grading, consulting students, etc. Make sure that your workload is balanced regarding teaching, research, and service (i.e. committee assignment, administrative duties), and most importantly, make sure your workload fits your needs and your career aspirations. The selection of the working environment is crucial in terms of your workload. For example, in my department, new faculty members do not teach in their first year as our focus is on research.

7.2.1.3 Equipment

Make sure you know availability and condition of equipment. If the equipment you need is not available, it is very important that you know, in detail, the prices of equipment you need. It is also a good idea to have two lists developed; essential and desirable. Then, during the negotiations, you can approach the discussion as a person that does not want everything up because you are flexible. Such flexibility could be appreciated, and you could gain in other areas, such as a higher salary, that may be more important for you and your family. Furthermore, you need to know if the available equipment is shared. If this is the case, then what is the policy about sharing. For example, we have an equipment sharing policy in my Department of Biomechanics since nobody owns any of the equipment we possess.

7.2.1.4 Space

This is very similar with the equipment negotiations. You need to know, in advance, what kind of space you need. Do not forget office space for your personnel. There is also essential and desirable space. As we mentioned above remember to ask about the policy of sharing if the space is shared with others.

7.2.1.5   Funds for personnel

You can request funds for students, technicians, postdocs, and even personal assistants if you are moving to a higher position. You should explore the expense of such personnel before you request these funds. Their costs vary based on location. In addition, a university may be more willing to give you more students than technicians or postdocs, as they prefer to increase enrollment in their degrees. Make sure you ask such questions. As a young faculty, a general suggestion is to hire students and technicians instead of postdocs, as the latter usually cost more.

7.2.1.6   Moving expenses

This can also be part of the negotiations. You can request such expenses for moving your household to the new location, several plane tickets, etc.

7.2.1.7   Family members

Another item you can request is help obtaining a job for your significant other. Many universities want to make sure that your entire family is well placed and pleased with their new environment. This will certainly enhance your productivity![1]

7.2.1.8   Myths about start-up funds and negotiations

Myth 1: You must negotiate

Negotiations are not mandatory. Remember that future employers want to hire you (Eberle, 2013). So, when they ask you what you want, you could be reasonable by being prepared and knowing your own worth. The more you negotiate, the more friction you create. Remember that you will see your future employers again (if everything goes right). Therefore, it is important to start and maintain a good relationship with them. At the same time, this does not mean that you should not negotiate, but there's a thin line that you do not want to cross. Thus, as we mentioned earlier, it is

---

[1] For my first job, I did not negotiate for any of these items mentioned here. This was a terrible mistake. My equipment was archaic. The most important piece of equipment (a force platform) that was given to me was in another space that I could use only over the weekends. I was given a 75% teaching load. No funds for personnel besides two teaching assistants, and I accepted without any negotiation the salary that was given to me. It is truly a miracle that I have accomplished all the things that I was able to do in this university when starting with such a handicap. Unfortunately, I was not taught about the importance of negotiating for my start-up package. I didn't even know that something like start-ups exist. I entered the academic world with complete naivety. Hopefully, you are reading this book and you are learning from my many mistakes!

extremely important to conduct a thorough search on what the university can offer (equipment, personnel, etc.) and be well prepared.

Myth 2: Negotiation is a disingenuous process

There is nothing wrong with negotiating. However, remember the thin line that I just mentioned. You will need to find a fit between your interests and their interests. There are certain factors that are not negotiable. For example, if the university is not able to provide the necessary equipment needed to conduct your research, look for another university that can provide it.

Myth 3: Negotiation really means asking for more money

Negotiating for money is not the only item to consider. You should also consider items such as workload, space, equipment, staff, vacation time, travel funds, and moving expenses.

Myth 4: Men are better at this than women

Negotiating is not gender specific. My experience has taught me that good negotiating skills is not a gender specific trade. Always keep the other party's interests in mind (e.g. the department's mission and vision), be well prepared, and remember the individual skills you bring to your working environment.

Myth 5: Employers want to give the lowest offer

Your future employer has performed a significant amount of work before arriving to the point to make you an offer. They want to hire you. They do not want to disappoint you with a bad offer, as they want you to be productive and pleased to work with them. Thus, do not assume that the employer seeks to provide you with the lowest offer. If you are not pleased with their offer, first be thankful, then request information on how they have arrived at this amount and if it is negotiable. Then act accordingly. Remember that you may get the offer of your dreams, but everybody could be unhappy with you before you even start.

7.2.1.9 Additional hints on start-up funds

Hint 1: Remember what I call the locker room effect.

People tend to resent those who make more money than them while having the same position. Make sure you keep everyone around you happy as academia requires team work.

Hint 2: Make sure you conduct a thorough search before you move to a new environment (state or private sectors) to learn as much as you can about your future employers.

Remember that some trustworthy people consider a handshake more than a contract,[2] while others do not even care about written contracts

---

[2] I consider this as the highest compliment that an administrator from another university said about me to a young faculty member that I hired a few years ago. I attribute this to my mother.

and will not deliver as promised. A very good example of the latter was illustrated in an article published in Science (Mervis, 2011). Dr. Kelly Suter was promised a $230,000 start-up package when she decided to move to a new university, but due to bureaucracy (and her gender as she claimed), the university administrators did not keep their promise and did not provide the funds required. Adding to her anxiety was the fact that she moved into this new faculty position just before her grant renewal. I strongly advise that you should not move into a new faculty position on your fourth year of a 5-year federal grant, where you probably need preliminary data to be added; move on your first year. Dr. Suter decided to file a lawsuit and eventually the university delivered the funds. This was after a major delay which affected her progress. Personally, I believe that filing a lawsuit is never a good solution since it affects both parties involved. You do not want to escalate the issue into that situation since this may lead to a very toxic environment. However, Dr. Suter was also under a lot of pressure. Probably, her mistake was moving into a new environment without conducting a thorough research on faculties, chairman, and everyone who's involved with that environment. Before you decide to move into a new faculty position, make sure you conduct a thorough evaluation of the people working in that environment (their work ethics, funding opportunities, culture, etc.).

7.2.1.10   *Additional hints on negotiating an agreement*

Negotiation occurs at many levels and is part of life. However, it is not a skill with which most people are familiar. Here are some hints on how to achieve a favorable negotiation.

Hint 1: Break the ice

Try to create a comfortable environment. It is very useful if you have some information handy about the other party. If you do not have any such information, while sitting in his/her office to start with the interview, try to scan the environment for clues that may help you acquire some knowledge about them. When you start your conversation bring up first the clue you identified: "Do you like soccer?" "Me too, I played in high school!" "What was your position?" etc. Then slowly move into speaking about your needs. I highly advise you to learn everything possible about the specific person with whom you intend on negotiating. Ask other people who know him/her, and find all the clues you can possibly identify on the internet. Almost everyone is exposed on social media, which makes it easier to gather information. These gathered clues will help strengthen your negotiation success by creating a comfortable environment in the beginning. Speaking about them will put them at ease and get them ready to listen. Since I mentioned social media, I also advise you to be extremely careful on what you share online. Your future employer will also scan you for similar clues and knowledge about you.

Hint 2: Listen and identify the need

Negotiating requires two parties that would like to reach a balanced agreement for their respective needs. So, start by making them feel that you really understand their problems. As an example, a student who is looking for a postdoc position should first "break the ice" as described above and then should ask about the requirements of the position to attain the specific information needed to relate experiences to qualifications. In general, "buy" first by carefully listening and identifying the needs. Then start "selling" yourself by explaining how well you can address these needs and what a great fit you are.

Hint 3: Deliver your solution

Once you identify their needs, address them immediately by delivering your solution based on your expertise and qualifications. Be specific and try not to drift away from your solution, as you may mention something that may weaken your negotiating agreement.

Hint 4: Wait for the agreement to come

Wait and do not rush it. Do not corner the other person. Propose your needs based on strong arguments and wait for the other person to respond by making sure you provide them with the necessary time they need to make their decision. Once you propose your solution, maintain silence. As soon as you have what you want, a desirable outcome, leave to avoid more talking that can create problems which may lead to a disagreement and a reversal of the outcome you just worked so hard to achieve.[3]

7.3   Presenting and teaching

There are many books on how to become a great teacher and an excellent presenter (see references at the end of the chapter). Therefore, my goal is not to list here skills such as how to make an exam or a syllabus. What I would like to present to you in this section is some personal advice in terms of teaching and presenting.

7.3.1   Personal hints

First, I believe that teaching and presenting go hand in hand. An effective teacher is also an engaging and effective presenter who not only uses audiovisual elements but also uses storytelling and even anecdotes. Below are some personal hints on becoming a strong teacher and presenter.

---

[3] I once had a brilliant but very talkative student. When he finished working with me, he applied towards several jobs. Usually my students are quite successful; however, this student faced multiple rejections because he was so talkative and created problems that were not present before.

Hint 1: Always be well prepared.

It is very important that you understand the material you present extremely well. If you present any data, make sure that you have compared them with data from the literature. The worst that can happen to you is to have results from human subjects which are so different that are only achievable by superhumans (this is a true story from a meeting that I was attending)! In terms of your classroom, make sure that you go over all your assigned readings and all the materials you have available before your lecture. You need to demonstrate that you are knowledgeable on the subject matter and you want to radiate confidence to your students.

Hint 2: Incorporate humor in your presentation.

Try to work on some jokes that you sprinkle through your lectures and presentations. If a joke generates a good reaction, maintain it for the future. I always like to observe stand-up comedians to learn how they try to engage their audience. Everybody loves a good joke and will certainly help you break the ice and get your audience more enthused. However, remember that a lecture or a scientific presentation is not stand-up comedy.

Hint 3: Dress well.

Even now, after almost 30 years of teaching, I dress at least business casual when I go to teach. Business casual for females is a combination of a skirt or dress slacks, blouse, sweater, twinset, jacket (optional), and hosiery (optional) with closed toe shoes. For males is a combination of dress slacks, a button-down shirt, dark socks, and dress shoes. For meetings or any other work-related functions, I dress traditional business. This attire for females is a combination of skirt suits or pantsuits with formal business blouses or tops, stockings, closed toe and heel leather shoes, and appropriate business accessories including a briefcase, a leather folder for pads of paper, and a conservative pen. For males is a combination of formal suit, tie, business shirt, upscale sports jackets with ties and a business shirt, leather dress shoes, appropriate conservative leather accessories such as briefcases, portfolios, and diaries.

Of course, many people will disagree with me on this topic and do not care about appearances especially nowadays. However, I am a strong believer that first impressions can take you far. You never know when you may meet a future employer or a collaborator. In addition, this is my way of demonstrating respect towards my students, my colleagues at a scientific meeting, the organizers of the meeting, etc.

Hint 4: Obey the rules of your presentation.

If you are given 50 min to talk, make sure that you do not go over the allotted time. Prepare well and practice multiple times. Adhere by all the rules given to you for your oral presentation or for your poster or for your class lecture. If you are teaching a class that spans multiple hours or a long workshop, give frequent breaks. I like to give a break every 45 min. Such breaks will decrease boredom that usually sets in after 50 min and will provide both a physical and mental time-out. My breaks are usually 10 min. I also make sure that I state this duration before I give a break. Otherwise, your audience will not know when to come back. I also start sharp after the expiration of the break without waiting for everybody to come back. This provides a sense of seriousness and structure which is necessary for long classes and workshops. Lastly, I always start strong (with examples or an interesting topic) after the break to recapture the attention of my audience. Therefore, I time my breaks in order to have something really interesting to say as soon as they are back. Many times, I also do a short recap to bring everything together in their minds and connect any lose dots.

Hint 5: Go early and test all equipment used.

You never know what can go wrong. I have seen the worst in my career regarding technology. However, the same can happen in your every week lectures or brief presentations. Thus, go early to decrease any added stress that can be produced by technology. You have enough stress already from your actual presentation. In addition, make sure that you have your presentation stored on different media such as your laptop but also on an external storage device or the cloud because you never know what you may face.

Hint 6: Be cordial in your answers.

If you will face questions, make sure that you are cordial and specific in your response. Do not engage in a conversation in front of a large audience as many people may not want to listen to multiple questions from the same individual, as they may have some questions of their own. Ask these individuals to find you after your lecture to discuss the matter further. If you do not know the answer to a question, acknowledge this and do not speculate. Being honest is always the correct approach.

If you are an attendee and you want to ask a question, be brief in your question as you are not the presenter. Finish your question with a question mark. In other words, do ask a question and not just make a statement. Ask one question, as this is not a conversation except if it is otherwise specified as part of a classroom or a lecture exercise. Be cordial and honest with your questions. Do not ask questions for which you already know the answers or ask questions so the rest of the audience will recognize that you are present! More experienced people than you will be able to discern this and you may be embarrassed.

Hint 7: Always be fair.

Never treat your lecture attendees or your students differentially. If you give one question to one person, you should not give more to another. If possible, your responses should also be of the same time length. As an instructor, always adhere to the guidelines that you presented the first day of your class. It is really important to explain to the students how their grade will be derived down to every single point. Your syllabus needs to be very specific and explain all procedures. Treat everybody equally on all situations (late assignments, missing exams, absences, etc.).

Hint 8: Examples, examples, examples.

You need to explain your material to your audience in such a fashion that they understand it. Provide multiple examples and illustrate your point very well. Make a habit to collect examples for your presentations from everywhere (i.e. seminars, meetings, even from movies). Personal stories carry even more weight. Examples can also be provided outside the classroom or the lecture hall in a form of additional readings or exercises that will require the participants to further explore the topic.

Hint 9: Engage your audience.

If you are teaching a class, ask questions to see if they understand the materials presented but also to engage them in critical thinking. Do they know of any other examples? Are they aware or can they think of any other ways that can utilize the materials presented? I personally like to ask questions to everybody, even the students who are shy and never talk. I try to learn everybody's name by taking roll before every class. Addressing them with their names makes them feel more comfortable in your presence.

In terms of science, there is nothing more important than enhancing critical thinking as we mentioned in previous chapters. Thus, my questions in my classes or in my reading clubs are thought provoking and not about description of materials. I never start a conversation by asking what is this paper about. I move straight into asking what is that you find interesting in this paper or what is that you identified as a major weakness or limitation. Another question that I really like is how a paper fits in the logical tree of the authors or you would modify the design if you did this experiment yourself. In terms of a scientific presentation, you may want to ask in the beginning of your lecture a question that requires your audience to raise their arms or do something that will engage their participation.

The above will give a sense to your audience that you are doing this presentation together and they are teaching you as much as you are teaching them! They are also presenters right there with you.

Hint 10: Avoid confrontations.

Always avoid confrontations, especially in front of others. If you feel that the conversation is escalating to the point of inappropriateness, take a time-out! In other words, leave and ask to revisit this point at a later time. Time-outs are very important not only in the sport that I played, basketball, but also in life, in general. When you return a graded exam to your students, do not engage immediately after class in conversations regarding the grades. My rule is to ask the students to come and find me on another day to discuss their disagreements in more detail. The students will come and find you in a much calmer state and the conversation will be much more amenable and civilized. In the same realm, always give your grades to the students at the end of the class; otherwise, their attention and participation will be affected.

Hint 11: The exams.

There is not a lot you can do to make an exam exciting and its time less stressful. However, I have found out that if you "dress up" a little, you can at least give a smile to the students. For example, put on a mustache or an eye-patch when you give the exams! I also like to start my exam with a little "confession" about myself. For example, I may tell them something like "I love to read theology." Then ask them to do the same on the first page of the exam. This relaxes them as they think of something that they really enjoy doing. In addition, I include some general words of wisdom or quotes from famous people on the first page of the exam and some poetry at the end. Some of my exams also have real-life scenarios to make them more exciting. In Vignette 7.1, I have included a few questions from one of my biostatistics exams to give you an idea. Lastly, I like to combine all possible means of questioning in my exams (e.g. multiple choice, fill in the blanks, essay, etc.). The literature (see Additional Readings) supports such an approach.

VIGNETTE 7.1 This test has a title. It is called: A "REAL"-LIFE EXPERIENCE

Imagine yourself sitting in your office when another graduate student comes running in looking for some help and exclaims, "I have a meeting with my advisor tomorrow and need some statistical questions answered!" Knowing that advisors demand correct answers, you educate this individual with clear and concise responses. The petrified student first describes the study. My study has one independent variable, length of exercise training regime, with four levels – 10, 20, 30, and 40 min in duration. My dependent variable is the number of hours an individual can exercise without stopping. I believe that people with longer training regimes should be able to exercise longer without stopping than those people with shorter training regimes. I individually tested 15 people per group. Here are the means and standard deviations:

10 min	20 min	30 min	40 min
0.78	2.0	2.4	2.6
(0.78)	(1.3)	(0.99)	(1.3)

1. Why can't I just run multiple *t*-tests to examine differences in group means? Why do I have to run a completely randomized one-way (single-factor) analysis of variance? (XX pts)
2. My advisor told me that running a single-factor analysis of variance requires meeting some assumptions. What are these assumptions and does my data meet these assumptions? (XX pts)
3. I wanted to select my alpha level, as just about every other researcher does, to equal 0.05, but my advisor suggested 0.025. How does adopting my advisor's suggested alpha level influence type I error, type II error, and power? (XX pts)

....

And continues like that.

Hint 12: You can always improve your teaching and presenting.

There are multiple ways to improve your teaching and presenting skills. In my career, I have used several techniques that have helped me enormously. Here are four that I consider the best:

- Peer-evaluation from more experienced colleagues
- Mid-term evaluations from my students
- Evaluations from my audience during a scientific meeting
- Recording myself and performing a self-evaluation .

Hint 13: Write a teaching philosophy statement.

It is not only important to have a teaching philosophy, but also to be able to write an excellent teaching philosophy statement, as it is required for most jobs in the academic market. Here is some advice regarding this task.

- You need to write a statement that is clear, readable, with no grammar and orthographical errors. Try also to be brief (no more than two pages).
- I recommend that you use a first-person approach, making it more personal and reflective. Make sure that you explain that you value teaching and you are committed to become an excellent teacher, including future pedagogical development plans. Demonstrate enthusiasm and do not present teaching as a burden to research.

- You need to present your student goals, as well as your teaching and assessment methods. Make sure that you write clearly how you deal with diversity and student differences in terms of learning capabilities.
- Make sure that you include precise descriptions of your disciplinary context and use detailed examples of your practice.
- Feature your strengths and accomplishments by using personal examples and demonstrating that you are a thoughtful instructor.

7.3.2   The poster

One frequent form of presentation is the poster presentation (Zielinska, 2011). Below I will provide you with some hints on how to generate an effective poster for your next scientific meeting. Some of these hints are also applicable in the generation of your slides for lectures.

Hint 1: Decrease the amount of text and increase the number of figures.

You need to think in figures. Can you use a figure or a picture to describe your methods, your results, your conclusions, etc.? In addition, try to avoid tables where numbers may be too difficult to read. Translate tables into bar graphs which are viewer friendly and much easier to be understood. Do not forget to label all axes in your figures. If you use text, make sure that you shorten your lines, you use bullets, gaps between lines, and most importantly, consider breaking your poster into three to four columns. In general, consider a ratio between graphs and texts that is at least equal to 50/50. However, a very good rule of thumb is to try to remove all text and see if your poster can stand alone just by using the figures that remain. If you have accomplished this, then you are on the right track.

Hint 2: I prefer to use left justification in a poster even though in grants I use full.

Left justification works better if you are standing in front of something that you are trying to read instead of having pages and pages of a grant in front of you as a reviewer. I never use center justification except in the Title of the poster.

Hint 3: You also need to consider the fonts you will use.

I prefer to use Sans Serif like Helvetica or Gill Sans for the text in the body of the poster and Serif for the titles. You can also try the other way around if you prefer that. Never use Comic Sans as they look quite unprofessional. Importantly, I recommend that you differentiate text from titles by giving each a different font. Consider also the size of your fonts. Try to use all of the space on your poster, eliminating any empty space. This is accomplished, not by adding more information, but by increasing the size of your fonts because, in this case, bigger will be better. Remember people will be standing in front of your poster, and they will try to read it. Not everybody has your perfect 20/20 vision. You also want to capture those who just walk by and just read your title, quickly. In general, I try to use 85 pt for the title, 44 pt for the headers, and 34 pt for the text in the body of the poster.

Hint 4: The proper usage of colors can hinder or enhance the quality of your presentation.

My advice is to use white as the background color or at least a color very close to white. For the text in the body of the poster, I prefer to use black or colors very close to black. This will give a more professional tone in your poster. You certainly need to avoid using primary colors on other primary colors such as reds on blues or reds on yellows. Remember also that many times colors may look quite different on your computer screen than when printed. Thus, print a small copy of your poster to check the colors.

Hint 5: The organization of your poster is also very important.

Many presenters place their conclusions at the end which is usually the bottom right corner of their poster. This will require many times that your audience to bend towards the floor in order to read them, even though most people will stay on eye level information neglecting anything below that. However, your conclusions are probably one of the first things that your audience will read. Therefore, I recommend that you place them on the top right corner of your poster. In general, keep more important and most read material on the top (i.e. introduction, hypotheses, key graph, conclusions). Another key element is to avoid any type of repetition and utilize your space wisely. For example, provide answers to your hypotheses in your conclusions instead of rewriting results or simply restating the significance of your study.

Hint 6: It is an advertisement of your work.

You always need to think that a poster is practically an advertisement of your work. However, it needs to be a presentation of substance and not a "Coca-Cola" poster. Your research will carry the substance. Thus, go to a meeting to present when you have something important to share with your peers. I also advise you to have a draft of the paper that is based on the information of the poster almost ready for submission. Remember, that as soon as you present your work, your ideas are exposed. Always print a color copy of your poster to check the layout, its readability from distance, and if it adheres with the poster rules of the meeting. At the meeting, you need to have available copies of your poster to share with individuals that were not able to be at your poster at the designated time of your presentation. This is very important because you will find yourself talking about your work multiple times during the scientific meeting. If you gave an oral presentation, prepare a short one-page handout to share with other scientists during similar conversations.

Hint 7: Practice, practice, practice.

Make sure you practice your poster multiple times with your mentor and your laboratory colleagues. However, remember that this is not an oral presentation. Thus, you need to practice what is called your elevator or 1-min speech. See later in the chapter for some hints about preparing such a speech.

7.3.3   Oral presentation

Several of the above hints also apply to the development of effective slides for oral presentations for a scientific meeting or classroom lectures. However, I have included below some additional and more specific hints for this purpose.

Hint 1: Remember the "determinants of the oral presentation."

1. Keep your graphs clear, even if the context is quite complex. For example, use bar graphs over graphs with multiple overlapping lines.
2. Use photos and images to help the audience remember something that you mention.
3. Include one point per slide and keep your presentation as one slide per minute.
4. Use as little text as possible and keep your text lines simple.
5. Follow the rules given to you by the organizers.

Hint 2: Your first slide is your title slide.

Your title slide should include the title of your presentation, your name, your affiliation, acknowledgments, and a visual as a hook. Acknowledging sponsors early is important, especially if they are in the audience as will make them feel pleased with their investment. You do not need to restate your name and title if someone else has presented you. You can go straight to your acknowledgments and to your hook.

Hint 3: Your hook slide.

If you have a separate slide as your hook slide or attention grabber, make sure this is your first slide after your title. The hook slide could include the reason for the research or the unanswered question or a surprising result. It provides momentum and energizes the audience. Make sure that it connects with your title, it is not highly technical, too long, overly promising, or text-heavy.

Hint 4: The map slide.

If you have a long presentation, you can use a map slide to provide a logical structure of your talk and allow the audience to keep track of time. You can reinsert this slide when you start with the other parts of your presentation to remind the audience of what is coming up next.

Hint 5: The story slides.

After the map slide, you include the story slides. The story slides should be connected. Your story should flow without being too complex or too general and superficial. A good presentation is like watching a movie with an excellent scenario and superb acting. At the end, the mystery should be solved! Avoid transitions between slides like fading as they distract from the story you are telling. Lead the audience based on logic and strong inference (see chapter one). You should also include brief titles in each slide that stress the point you are making. Remember to have one point per slide. I recommend that you have your title on a black background with white text, while the rest of the slide is exactly the opposite. Regarding the text, do not go above 50 words for a story slide that you will spend 1.5 min speaking.

Hint 6: At the end, you need to include your summary slide.

In this slide, you deliver on what you promised. Thus, you need to connect it back to your title and your hook slide. I personally prefer to provide also a take-home message that the audience can remember and even utilize in their lives to make it more personal. In addition, I provide some hints on what is coming up next based on my logical tree. This will leave the audience with the feeling of wanting to hear me again because the sequel will be equally exciting! These last two points will also provide the audience with great opportunities for questions without having to recall your entire presentation. I recommend that you avoid finishing up with your limitations but include them within the story slides.

Hint 7: The thank-you slide.

I always finish with a thank you slide towards the organizers of my talk even though several books on how to present recommend against it. On that slide, I usually include some pictures of my environment in Nebraska to give a more personal note to my presentation. I include a thank you slide because I believe that cordiality and gentility are fundamental in life.

Hint 8: Have a drink on the podium.

Always have something to drink on your podium as your vocal chords could be stressed. However, keep it as far away as possible from the computer you are using because an accident could be devastating! This advice comes from someone who is a very clumsy scientist! In addition, avoid having coffee as your drink of choice as coffee could make you even more jittery and result in a pointer that moves even more erratically in your hands. This may give the impression that you are too nervous when you want to portray the exact opposite that you are confident presenter.

7.4   Being an administrator

At some point in your career, you may be required to step up into an administration position. This could happen for multiple reasons, such as seeking a new challenge in your career or an elevation in salary or you may want to influence governance in your environment or even because you want to avoid someone else becoming your boss. Several years ago, I became a Chair of a department that I developed, and even more recently, a Director of a Center as well as an Assistant Dean with major responsibility the guidance of an Academic Division. During these times, I read several books on how to be a successful administrator and received some training. I have included some of the books that I read in my list of suggested readings at the end of this chapter. From these readings, but mostly from my own personal experiences, I am listing below several hints on how to become a successful administrator.

7.4.1 Hiring

One of the most important aspects of your job will be to hire excellent staff and faculty members. This starts with writing strong job descriptions and position announcements that include the type of employee you really need and your specific expectations, as well as the type of supporting materials that should be submitted to help you derive to the best decision possible. Furthermore, your interviews need to be well organized, allowing you to gather all important information you need to make your final decision. Remember that the hiring of faculty members, who also receive a positive tenure decision, will turn them into your colleagues for many years.

Hint 1: The materials you request

When I seek to hire a faculty member, I request a variety of materials beyond the standard letters of references, transcripts, and resume. These may include the following: statements of a candidate's philosophy of teaching, research, and service; a sample syllabus or final exam; a faculty development plan for teaching and research over the next 5 years; a set of specific aims for the first grant that they will write if they get the position; and suggestions over one book every student in our discipline should read. Such materials will allow for a better judgement of the potential of your new faculty member.

Hint 2: Be specific in your job description

Clearly indicate in the job description certain important items, such as the starting date of the position, any required qualifications, the type of the position you are hiring (i.e. tenure-track Assistant Professor), proper contact information, deadlines for submission of materials (make sure that these deadlines do not fall on weekends or holidays), and how the materials should be submitted. Such specific information will eliminate many problems during the hiring process.

Hint 3: The search committee

After you assemble the search committee responsible for the position you are advertising, make sure you explain clearly to them the type of the individual the department or the college would like to hire. Request that they utilize a ranking system for all the candidates to maintain a written record of their recommendation. In their ranking system, they can include scores for all the credentials submitted and the qualifications required in the job description. I usually provide them with an example, but I also allow them the freedom to develop their own tools. Such materials will help you justify the decision process to higher administration. Provide to your search committee sufficient time to review all materials and explain well the purpose of their on-campus interview with the candidates selected.

Hint 4: The on-campus interview

Clearly explain to the candidate the type of presentation you would like them to provide (i.e. research seminar, teaching a class) as well as the length of their presentation. Provide them with the opportunity to meet with other faculty, students, technicians, research associates, and staff. Eventually, you will request that all these individuals will provide you with feedback on the candidates. Again, I utilize a ranking type of feedback where I welcome grading on the candidate's qualifications, as well as comments on the grades provided. This allows everybody to participate in the hiring process in a very democratic fashion. I also try to meet with the candidate both during an interview in my office and in a more casual fashion having dinner. Regarding the interview questions that I use, I refer you to the previous chapter where I provided a long list of such questions.

7.4.2   Firing

Letting someone go is also part of the job. However, it is the most difficult part. It requires immense attention to detail and extreme caution. Here are some hints regarding this painful experience for all parties involved.

Hint 1: Get advice

Make sure that you discuss the situation with higher administration and your human resources office. Get them involved in the process and incorporate all advice they have for you. Gather all information they ask you to obtain and ensure that they are always in agreement with your actions. Have their agreement in writing.

Hint 2: The timing

My advice is to act sooner than later. Giving repeated chances to unsuccessful individuals is not merciful but misleading. You also need to maintain good documentation on everything that has been done, while you also follow the university's internal procedures to the letter. During the actual dismissal, be brief without revealing more than you need. At that time, you need to be honest and respectful.

7.4.3 *Mentoring faculty members*

I have already dedicated an entire section of a previous chapter on mentoring. However, here I would like to mention one additional tool that I use regarding the mentoring of faculty members from the perspective of a Chair. This is the Individual Development Plan (IDP); see Vignette 7.2 for a sample IDP. An IDP can also be used for the mentoring of postdocs. The IDP provides a planning process that identifies professional development needs as well as career objectives. It allows you to make specific steps in your career rather than going through a "random walk." IDPs can also serve as tools to help facilitate communication between junior faculty and their mentor/chairperson. An IDP can help junior faculty identify

- Long-term career goals they would like to pursue and tools to meet these goals.
- Short-term needs for improving current performance.

The development, implementation, and revision of the IDP requires a series of steps to be conducted by the junior faculty member, and then discussed with his/her mentor/chairperson. These steps are:

Step 1. Conduct a skills assessment: The junior faculty member conducts an assessment of their strengths, weaknesses, and skills; then asks their mentor/colleague to review their skills assessment with the mentee.

Step 2. Complete the IDP: The junior faculty member states their career goals and writes their Annual IDP. Make sure you incorporate SMART goals that are Specific, Measurable, Action-oriented, Realistic, and Time-bound.

Step 3. Implement the IDP: The junior faculty member sets an appointment with their mentor/chairperson; discusses the IDP with their mentor/chairperson; implements the steps in the IDP; and periodically reviews progress with their mentor/chairperson.

Note for the faculty member: Make this appointment with your mentor/chairperson separate from other lab meetings. An environment away from the lab will eliminate distractions. During this meeting be positive saying something like: "I've really enjoyed my last year in the lab, and I feel I've made progress on project X ..." Do not attempt to share the entire IDP and prepare a concise written outline for the meeting. Lastly, be prepared to negotiate for aspects of the IDP that you did not complete.

VIGNETTE 7.2   Sample IDP

STEP 1: SKILLS ASSESSMENT

Assess your strengths, weaknesses, and skills.
     Evaluate your skills and abilities in the following areas:

General Research Skills

Designing program evaluations/studies	1	2	3	4	5
Analytical skills	1	2	3	4	5
Problem-solving/troubleshooting	1	2	3	4	5
Creativity/developing new research directions	1	2	3	4	5

Teaching Skills

One-on-one teaching	1	2	3	4	5
Small group teaching	1	2	3	4	5
Large group presentation	1	2	3	4	5

Professional Skills

Grant writing skills	1	2	3	4	5
Oral presentation skills	1	2	3	4	5
Manuscript writing skills	1	2	3	4	5
Mentoring skills	1	2	3	4	5
Being a mentee	1	2	3	4	5

Leadership and Management Skills

Leading and motivating others	1	2	3	4	5
Budgeting	1	2	3	4	5
Managing projects and time	1	2	3	4	5
Organizational skills	1	2	3	4	5

Interpersonal Skills

Getting along with others	1	2	3	4	5
Communicating clearly in writing	1	2	3	4	5
Communicating clearly in conversation	1	2	3	4	5

5 = Highly proficient.

1 = Needs improvement.

Once you have completed the skills assessment, set up a
meeting with your mentor/chairperson to discuss.

STEP 2: WRITE AN ANNUAL IDP THAT EVALUATES YOUR PROGRESS DURING THE LAST YEAR AND SETS GOALS FOR THE UPCOMING YEAR.

Fill out the Annual IDP. Your IDP is an evolving document as
needs and goals change throughout your career. The objective

is to set clearly defined career goals. Your IDP will assist you with creating a strategy for building upon current strengths and skills over the upcoming year while also providing you with a plan to address areas that need further development.

Objectives of an Annual IDP:

- Create an annual outline that will help you achieve long-term career goals.
- Establish target dates for the completion of various training or skills improvement opportunities.
- Set goals and sub-goals for the next year, including a discussion of how you will spend your time.
- Define in detail the strategy you plan to implement in order to acquire the skills and strengths needed (e.g. courses, technical skills, teaching, supervision) along with an anticipated time frame for acquiring those skills and strengths.

Annual IDP

Academic Year

Faculty Member

Today's Date:

Current academic title/rank:

Career and Professional Goals

What are your professional goals for the upcoming year?

What are your long-term career goals (3–5 years)?

What are the motivating factors for pursing these particular goals?

Are there special circumstances or barriers that may make it more challenging to achieve your goals for the upcoming year?

What were your main goals for the past year?

Which of the goals (mentioned above) did you meet? If you did not meet a goal, why?

Time Management

By your best estimate, how did you allocate your time during the past year?

Percentage of time spent on teaching, training, or mentoring others

Percentage of time spent on research and/or creative work

Percentage of time spent on service/administration
Percentage of time spent on other duties
How, if at all, will you change this time distribution in
the coming year?
Development of General Research Skills
What further research-related skills do you
need to acquire to be successful in this step of your
career and in the next step? What will you do during the next year to improve in this area?
Development of Teaching Skills
What further teaching-related skills do you
need to acquire to be successful in this step of your
career and in the next step? What will you do during the next year to improve in this area?
Development of Professional Skills
What further development do you need in the
areas of grant writing, oral presentation of your
work, manuscript writing, mentoring, or being a
better mentee? What will you do during the next
year to improve in these areas?
Development of Leadership and Management Skills
What further development do you need in the
areas of leadership, budgeting, time management,
project management, and organization? What will
you do during the next year to improve in these
areas?
Development of Interpersonal Skills
What further development do you need in this
area? What will you do during the next year to
improve in this area?
Development of Your CV
Update your CV and attach it to this IDP.
Final Goal Setting and Prioritizing
Overall, what goals will receive your top priority for the coming year? Create a monthly timeline
for fulfilling these goals and attach it to this IDP.

STEP 3: IMPLEMENT YOUR PLAN

1. Put your plan into action. Put your IDP that is somewhere easy to find and read over on a regular basis
to check your progress.

2. Each professional goal should be broken down into its smaller, accomplishable sub-goals, steps, or "deliverable," with specific dates for completing each of the sub-goals. The smaller goals should ultimately lead to accomplishment of the final goal. For example:

  Major goal: Submit a paper for publication
  Completion date: March 2019

  i. Sub-goal #1: Complete data analysis, figures, and outline.
  Completion date: October 2018
  ii. Sub-goal #2: Complete the Introduction section.
  Completion date: November 2018
  iii. Sub-goal #3: Complete the Discussion section.
  Completion date: December 2018

3. Revise and modify the plan as necessary. The plan will need to be modified as circumstances and goals change. One of the challenges of implementation is to remain flexible and open to change.

4. Plan to set a monthly meeting with your mentor/ chairperson to review and discuss your IDP. Be sure to prepare a written outline for the discussion. For example, create a prioritized list of the most important items you wish to discuss.

5. Revise your IDP on the basis of these discussion.

7.4.4   Running the department

There are many important items that you need to consider as you run the department (or the college being a Dean), and below I have included some hints on how effectively to do so.

Hint 1: Be a leader.

One of the best advices that were given to me when I became a Chair was from a senior well-respected faculty member from a prestigious university who described to me who was the best Chairperson he ever had. In this description, it was clear to me that this individual was the one who led by example his/her faculty members. The effective Chairperson was also successful in running a research team, publishing and writing grants, and being a productive faculty member himself. In addition, the effective Chairperson was in the classroom teaching; less than the other faculty members but still teaching a course.

I have followed this example as well as I could. Practically, such actions will demonstrate that you, as the Chairperson, are still there in the "trenches" with the other faculty members. Interestingly, the above advice was also given to me if I wanted to become a Dean or a Vice Chancellor from successful Deans and Vice Chancellors. Never forget your research and your teaching to maintain the respect of your faculty members, as they will recognize that you are still one of them. Then the question becomes one of balancing all acts. This is certainly difficult but not impossible. It requires discipline and excellent time management skills. Time management was presented in a previous chapter but here I also want to mention that you can achieve these goals by dedicating certain times during the day for your research and teaching. However, try to teach a course that you really enjoy teaching that does require a tremendous amount of preparation. Regarding your research, you may have to lead a smaller team, and thus, it will be important to hire excellent students and postdocs.

Hint 2: It is the little things.

Many times, they are the little things that improve the effectiveness of running a department. Here are some that I consider quite useful:

- Publicly recognize success of your faculty members. I do so in our Departmental Seminar Series, in our social functions, and in our faculty meetings.
- Reward productivity. I have worked with the University's Foundation to reward faculty members monetarily when they receive federal grants.
- Have faculty meetings that do not run long and maintain collegiality. If my faculty meetings last longer than an hour, I make sure that I apologize to my faculty members.
- Confront rumors head-on.
- Implement an annual theme that carries into your Departmental Seminar Series. Such a theme could be decided during your annual retreat in the beginning of the year. I always have such a retreat in an off-campus location to organize the entire year with my faculty members.
- Be transparent in your decision-making process and involve everybody through voting. This will allow your faculty members to work more as a team and not as individuals.
- Keep clear records and share budget decisions with your faculty members. Your budget should always be tightly connected to the mission and vision of your institution and your department. The way you will handle any indirect cost or salary savings that will come back to your department, should be of reinvesting back to your unit in an extremely fair and transparent way. You should reward productivity but also invest in potential.

- Revisit every year your mission and vision statements with all your faculty members and update them if necessary. I do so in my annual retreat in beginning of the academic year.
- Social events can help more than you think. My department is fortunate to have its own building. However, I ask everybody to have lunch in our break area and socialize. I also have a coffee every month with every single one of my faculty members.
- Perform evaluations to improve your environment. Every year I perform an evaluation of our Center members which practically entails our entire department. In addition, I meet once a year with every single student who is funded and works in our building. They have 15 min to discuss with me any problems that they may have or provide suggestions to improve our environment.
- Write effective annual evaluations for your faculty members. I spend a significant amount of time in writing my faculty members annual evaluations because I want to make sure that I provide constructive criticism. In my meetings with them, I am honest in explaining in writing what I expect from them, the areas that they perform well, as well as the areas that need improvement.
- Mentoring, mentoring, mentoring. In addition to the IDP, I always connect my faculty members with successful senior faculty members outside of our department that can help them with their careers. For our seminar series, I make every effort to bring excellent scientists and academicians, and I make sure that my faculty members have sufficient time with them to receive advice and feedback for their work.

7.5   The social factor

Being a successful scientist, academician, and investigator, requires one to be able to interact with others, network, collaborate, and socialize in an effective manner. Unfortunately, many times, scientists do not develop such skills because of the nature of their work: long hours in the laboratory working ascetically on data and writing manuscripts and grant proposals. Such isolation is necessary but could also hinder the development of your career. In this section, I provide you with some advice and hints to improve in this area in which I feel all scientists struggle including myself.

7.5.1   Friend-raising versus fund-raising

One of the most influential papers I read in this area was a profile of a very successful scientist, Dr. Antonio Giordano (Pain, 2007). Giordano is an Italian and American oncologist, pathologist, geneticist, researcher, professor, and writer. In his career, he was quite successful in attaining private funding. Private funding is completely different from federal funding, as you usually do not have to write grant proposal but you need to interact with donors and convince them of the importance and quality of your research. Giordano mainly received his private funding from "Sbarro." Sbarro is a U.S.-based chain of fast-food restaurants that is found in every mall, airport, and food court. The profile article (Pain, 2007) of Giordano states the following:

> As Giordano began to envision a research institute of his own, he got lucky. His wife to-be, whom he met during his time at Cold Spring Harbor, lived in the same New York neighborhood as the owners of Sbarro, a U.S.-based chain of fast-food restaurants that sells pizza and Italian dishes. Giordano soon encountered fellow Neapolitan Mario Sbarro and after almost a year of Sunday morning walks on Long Island won from him an initial donation of about $1 million to create the Sbarro Institute for Cancer Research and Molecular Medicine. Sbarro says he was impressed by Giordano, particularly his vision of 'creating an environment where talented [young] people ... could work together ... free of bureaucracy'.

I believe that Giordano created his own luck rather than being lucky. He was a successful scientist before he even met Sbarro. He has already developed a 10-person laboratory that studied cell cycle and cancer research using National Institutes of Health (NIH) funds that he received through his hard work. He also worked as a postdoc under the Nobel Prize winner James Watson at Cold Spring Harbor Laboratory, which provided him with remarkable experience. After his postdoc experience, he had started an outstanding career with several important findings in cancer-based research. He was an established scientist with a vision to change the world. Therefore, when he met Sbarro, he was well prepared and was able to deliver a specific message: "I am good, and if you provide me with more funds, I will be even better." The article does not describe well how exactly he met Sbarro; maybe through a party. It is common in the United States to throw neighborhood parties at least once a year, and it is possible that Giordano met Sbarro in such a party or maybe it was an Italian event as they were both Italians. What is important, though, is that you have to go to these events and social gatherings. Giordano probably went to one of these social gathering events and started introducing himself. Then, he probably started introducing his work through his 1-min speech and its impact on the cancer field. Sbarro did not open his checkbook immediately. It took a year until Sbarro decided to offer $1 million to help

Giordano achieve his dream. *This is what I call friend-raising, while other people call it fund-raising.*

However, Giordano did not stop there. The article (Pain, 2007) also states the following:

> To retain control of his private money, Giordano felt he needed to break free from the university's authority. But he also wanted the university's administrative support and infrastructure to keep non-research costs minimal. Convincing Temple to go along was not easy. In fact, in 1994, Giordano moved his lab to Thomas Jefferson University, also in Philadelphia, where he was offered an agreement that included the university matching Sbarro's donation. "After 2 years, my lab had tripled in number of people and space," Giordano says. But nearly a decade later, in 2002, Giordano returned to Temple after securing, in his words, "complete independence" in administering the funds, staff, research programs, and patent rights.

Giordano maneuvered himself quite effectively. Since Temple University refused Giordano's propositions, he decided to move to Thomas Jefferson University to break free from Temple's authority. He was able to receive better offers from Thomas Jefferson University where they offered to match all the private funds he received. *This proves that private funding provides tremendous amount of leverage.* Due to the amount of funds he received, his work tripled in just 2 years. This immediately proved his worth to his donor, as he delivered quite quickly on his promises through his hard work. After establishing an excellent career and earning national recognition, he went back to Temple University that recognized Giordano's value. He negotiated and attained complete independency. Sbarro continued helping him as he provided another $200,000 a year for 3 years as seed money. By 2007, the year of the publication of the article in *Science*, Giordano had raised $3 million in private funding, supplementing about $27 million that he and other investigators at his Sbarro Institute had obtained through federal and state grants. It is quite important to stress that Giordano continued working hard proving himself to his donor, receiving significant federal funding and elevating his environment.

Giordano is really an excellent example of a scientist that is engaged in the community to raise funds, practices friend-raising to support his environment, and diversifies his funding portfolio by adding private funds. Almost every scientist focuses on obtaining federal funds and then they work hard to renew them and maintain them. However, it has become more difficult to retain your federal grants. If you lose them, you may have to let go of your students, lab technicians, and postdocs. You may even lose your laboratory space and be forced to leave your institution. Giordano shows you another way where you diversify your portfolio by obtaining both private and federal funds. However, private funding requires that you get out of your laboratory (and your house) and socialize/network.

7.5.2   The steps to private funding and friend-raising

I had an experience quite similar to Giordano's. I was able to obtain a $6 million private donation to construct an entirely new building for biomechanics research in my university. The Biomechanics Research Building is the only research building on my university's campus and one of the world's first buildings dedicated to biomechanics research. This 23,000-square-foot building opened in 2013, and I moved my research team of 25 scientists into this state-of-the-art unique research environment. However, subsequent growth resulted in the Biomechanics Research Building currently housing over 70 faculty members, staff, and students, as well as being the home of the University of Nebraska at Omaha, Department of Biomechanics, and the Center for Research in Human Movement Variability. Therefore, I was able to raise another $12 million to expand the building by 30,000 square feet. This expansion will be ready by August of 2019. Below I describe the steps that I followed to make this happen.

7.5.2.1   Develop a good relationship with the University's Foundation

It is very important to develop a good relationship with the University's Foundation (if you are in a university) and private sector's foundation (if you work in private sector). The foundation already has a network of available donors and their goal is to actually raise funds. You really want to help them achieve their goals. They need to know you as a person, and they need to know your research.

7.5.2.2   Establish yourself in your own environment and good things will happen

When I first joined my university, nobody knew about me or my discipline. The word "biomechanics" was unknown in my university and even in my state. Therefore, I needed first to establish myself in my own environment before I could move forward for state and national recognition. This is done only through hard work; publications, grants, and everything else we already discussed. After I have established myself in my own environment, I was selected by my institution to attend a University of Nebraska Foundation event in Lincoln. Importantly, only one professor was selected by each Nebraska university. I was the one chosen by my institution. At that event, I had the opportunity to give a speech and talk about my achievements. Donors were invited to that event by the Foundation who wanted to raise funds to support deserving research. At the event, I went with added "ammunition." I brought with me my collaborator and excellent surgeon, Dr. Iraklis Pipinos, to enhance the credibility of my research and demonstrate its impact to society. We also provided the attendees with posters of the presentation and our annual biomechanics newsletter. At the social function that followed, I gave several 1-min speeches of my research to attendees of the event. Our presentation and ability to engage the attendees caught the eye of the President of the University as well as members of the Foundation. As a result, I was invited again to represent my institution during a second annual event at Palm Springs California. I gave the same presentation (this time without my collaborator though), but I also included at the end my vision of a building dedicated to biomechanics research. Ruth and Bill Scott were in the audience and in their words "felt in love with my message." Soon after, their son John Scott visited my laboratory and realized that we have performed amazing feats with truly limited resources. As an example, our current building manager had a closet as his office and patients used to change in the toilets of our recreation facilities. The Scott family decided to fund our building. Over the years also funded a professorship, fellowships for doctoral students, and even a mechanism to reward productivity among my department's faculty. They have practically treated me like a son, and I have worked even harder to make them proud of their investment in me. I have also received private funds from other donors that contributed to the current expansion of our building. Their contributions are now more that $4 million. Many of these donors are actually friends of the Scott family and were brought to our cause by them!

7.5.2.3   *Work in your message and your 1-min speech*

Your message needs to be clear and easy to be understood by everybody. This needs to be the case for your presentation to potential donors but even more importantly for your 1-min or "elevator" speech of your research to improve the impact of your work. This short speech will be given many times in social functions and gatherings. You need something similar to this when you stand in front of your poster in a scientific meeting. The goal of your 1-min speech is to stimulate interest. You want to give just enough; they can always ask for more. You also need to use familiar words and concepts. For example, it is better to use "wiring" than "microcircuitry." Here are some hints to develop your 1-min speech.

Hint 1: Think of your communication goals.

Examples of such goals are to increase understanding of what research is, to improve understanding of the value of research to the community, to enhance knowledge of research done here, to increase funding for science, to obtain funding for your own science, and to dialog with the community to better understand their beliefs regarding science.

Hint 2: Make sure you understand your audience.

Consider who are they and why should they care, what do they value, what keeps them up at night, how can you show you understand or empathize with their interests or needs, what angle will resonate most with them, and what might they be hesitant to hear.

Hint 3: Consider your "take-home" message.

Consider what is needed to deliver an effective take-home message. If it will require some background, then the key is to introduce *just enough*, especially if the topic is unfamiliar to your audience. Make sure that you do not talk like a scientist by avoiding jargon. Limit what you say by having one point in your take-home message and certainly no more than two.

Hint 4: Try to tell a story.

Telling a story is a powerful way to connect with your audience. As true for every story, it needs a beginning, a middle, and an end. The shorter the story, the better it is (Olson, 2009). The Beginning is an introduction of your topic with a couple of background statements. The Middle needs to create conflict, tension, and turn your science into a story. The End will provide the resolution and the rationale. Consider using the "And, But, Therefore" technique as described by Olson (Olson, 2009) and illustrated in the two examples below (Vignette 7.3).

VIGNETTE 7.3 EXAMPLES OF 1-MIN SPEECHES USING THE "AND, BUT, THEREFORE" TECHNIQUE

Example 1: The epidemic of obesity in adults and children is increasing our present and future healthcare costs. *And* we have proven that weight loss can prevent obesity-linked diseases like diabetes. *But* strategies that require changing behavior aren't easy to implement in a community-based clinic. *Therefore,* we are developing technology strategies that can be used in small town clinics to better prevent diabetes in youth and adults.

Example 2: My mother is 85 years old and has fallen many times. In general, falls in older adults is costing our healthcare system billions. *And* we know that when you get old the way you walk is different. *But* we still have not used this information to prevent falls. *Therefore,* in my research I am building devices that you can wear, and we develop simple movement based therapies to improve the way old people walk and keep them from falling and be safe.

7.5.2.4 *Delivering your 1-min speech*

One of the best examples of delivering a 1-min speech is from a movie called *Working Girl*. In this movie, Tess (played by Melanie Griffith and nominated for an Oscar) "gatecrashes" Oren Trask's (played by Philip Bosco) daughter's wedding to pitch her plan of a merger deal. She delivers her 1-min speech through a quick dance with Mr. Trask accomplishing her goal of setting up a meeting with him. Her delivery is absolutely marvelous and has the following characteristics. She is relaxed. No matter how important Mr. Trask is, she thinks that he is just a person. She is calm in her delivery. She takes a moment to think through what she wants to say. Her story has a beginning, a middle, and an end (see previous section). She also states who she is, what she does, why she is there, and why Mr. Trask should care about this.

From this example and my personal experiences, I am listing below few hints on how to deliver your 1-min speech.

- Be sure to be relaxed when you deliver your 1-min speech because whoever you are delivering that speech to is just a human being like you.
- Take a good breath and then start talking. State your name clearly and indicate your status (e.g. student, postdoc, professor). Mention what laboratory or university you work in.
- Then deliver your 1-min research speech using the "And, But, Therefore" technique. Make sure that you frame your work with the big picture: what you're interested in, how you approach it, and how it got you an invite to this event.
- Look the other person in the eye as you speak. If the angle is bad, pull out your chair slightly so that you can address them face-on. However, don't glare like a vulture, just make eye contact. In addition, make sure that you "check in" often to see if his/her face registers understanding, engagement, or a strong desire to ask a question.
- Pause if there seems to be a question brewing. Finish up by connecting what you've said back to the guest's interests or work. When you're done, stop talking and smile a natural smile. He/she might ask a question or just nod and shift his/her glance to the next person at the table or in the room, indicating that it's time for them to give their own introductions.

7.5.2.5 *Be passionate about your work*

I cannot stress enough how important it is to be passionate about your work when you are presenting or speaking to any potential's donors. You need to truly engage them and leave a long-lasting impression. You will never receive funds from your first meeting. All you need to do is create awareness about your problems, a potential friendship, and a strong memory of you and your work.

7.5.3   Networking

When you start a new job, it is very important to also start your network of friends and collaborators. Never forget to always friend-raise. This should also be the case when you attend scientific meetings. Below I have included some advice on how to improve your networking abilities.

7.5.3.1   Entering a room

When you are invited to or attend an event, it is really the manner in which you engage the rest of the people in the room (McCammon, 2011). President Clinton is still considered the best in entering a room and engaging the crowds. He practically owned the room because he was curious. He entered the room with curiosity. He wanted to talk to people and would totally engage them. He asked and remembered their names. The lessons from President Clinton are as follows: don't be aimless, don't be casual, and don't be flippant. Let your audience know they're important and that you're there because you have a message to give them.

If you are wearing a name tag, make sure it is located on your right shoulder at eye level. When you shake hands, wait for the person in a higher position of authority to be the first one to extend a hand. Among equals, older age extends first. Among genders, the lady always initiates. When you shake hands, make sure that you look the other person in the eye. Always use your right hand with a firm but not crushing grip which last for 2–3 s. However, always follow the lead of the superior person. Be aware of your other hand and always shake with an up and down motion.

7.5.3.2   Minimize uneasiness

To minimize uneasiness and build confidence, use these hints.

Hint 1: Network in small chunks.

Set a maximum of two carefully chosen events a month, ideally at your highest energy time of day. When I first moved to Omaha, I purchased opera season tickets. I used to go early before the opera starts, sit at the bar, have a drink, and try to engage people. If you don't know anyone in town, you have to do something. I chose opera, not only because I enjoy it, but also because you usually can meet quite interesting people.

Hint 2: Arrive early.

Entering an uncrowded room is less unnerving than a noisy one, where most people are already conversing. The rehabilitation social evening at the Society for Neuroscience annual meeting is usually attended by several successful senior scientists. I started attending this social the first time that I went to the meeting. I always went there early and talked to whoever walked in after me. I introduced myself and gave my 1-min speech to many individuals.

Hint 3: Go with a friend and preferably someone who can introduce you to several people.

If you are shy and you have a hard time engaging with the crowd, then you can invite a friend to keep you company and help you to make the first crucial steps in meeting at least a couple of other individuals.

Hint 4: Use safe "starters" to start your conversations.

Such starters include asking about their current job, why they chose this event, or what other groups they belong to. Seek topics of mutual interest, such as that gathering's focus. If you can offer information about anything that is mentioned, then make a note of this and follow up promptly. For every event you attend, gather business cards from people who are interesting to you and relate to your work and send them a note after the meeting showing your gratitude and thankfulness. Save all those business cards and send them wishes for the Holidays.

Hint 5: Choose smaller gathering where you can engage with fewer scientists.

I met two of my major collaborators, Drs. Pipinos and Oleynikov, at a social gathering in a friend's house. I have published over 40 papers with Dr. Pipinos, while I collaborated with Dr. Oleynikov for more than a decade. I initially gave them my 1-min speech which got them totally engaged. We end up conversing for hours creating, wonderful collaborations.

7.5.3.3   *Following-up*

I always follow up with the connections that I made during networking events with a note. You can certainly send an email but sending a handwritten letter or a card is unique and makes it special (Painter, 2011). Handwriting is rare nowadays, and even if it is bad, it is like showing your face. If you decide to use a handwritten note, find a nice paper or stationary instead of writing on a notebook sheet. Make sure you properly address the envelope, as a personal note or letter is like a "gift-wrapped thought."

Start your letter with "Dear (first name)" and end with "Truly," "Fondly," or whatever fits. In between, you can say that you hope they are doing well. Continue with some information about what you have been doing with an emphasis on events that mean something to your recipient. It is fine to ask questions, as a letter is like a conversation. When my university's Chancellor wants to congratulate someone, he also prefers sending a personal note or a letter. He will start his letter with "My dearest friend Nick" instead of "Dear Nick" and will finish with "Always your friend John." Lastly, I recommend that you use a fountain pen to generate a nice script.

References

Eberle, S. (2013). Let's make a deal. *The Scientist*, 2, 63–65.

McCammon, R. (2011). How to enter a room. *Entrepreneur*, August 18–19.

Mervis, J. (2011). Suit seeks redress for a start-up package gone sour. *Science*, 333, 24–25.

Olson, R. (2009). *Don't Be Such a Scientist*. Washington, DC: Island Press.

Pain, E. (2007). Dr. Hustle sells his dream for Italian medical research. *Science*, 316, 1118–1119.

Painter, K. (2011). Before your write of snail mail, make it personal. *USA Today*, August 11.

Zielinska, E. (2011). Poster perfect. *The Scientist*, 9, 55–57.

Additional Readings

Babcock, L., Laschever, S. (2007). *Women Don't Ask: The High Cost of Avoiding Negotiation-and Positive Strategies for Change*. New York: Bantam Publication.

Blaser, B., Editor (2010). *Career Trends: Building Relationships*. The American Association for the Advancement of Science. Washington, DC. Available online at: sciencecareers.org/booklets

Blaser, B., Editor (2010). *Career Trends: Running Your Lab*. The American Association for the Advancement of Science. Washington, DC. Available online at: sciencecareers.org/booklets

Brown, F.G. (1983). *Principles of Educational and Psychological Testings*. 3rd Edition. New York: Holt, Rinehart and Winston.

Buller, J.L. (2006). *The Essential Department Chair*. Bolton, MA: Anker Publishing.

Cottrell, D. (2002). *Monday Morning Leadership*. Dallas, TX: Cornerstone Leadership Institute.

Davis, B.G. (2009). *Tools for Teaching*. San Francisco: Jossey-Bass Publication.

Deluca, M.J., Deluca, N.F. (2006). *Perfect Phrases for Negotiating Salary and Job Offers*. New York: McGraw-Hill Publication.

Fisher, R., Patton, B.M., Ury, W.L. (1992). *Getting to Yes: Negotiating Agreement without Giving in*. 2nd Edition. Boston, MA: Houghton Mifflin Harcourt.

Goodyear, G.E., Allchin, D. (1998). Statements of teaching philosophy. In M. Kaplan & D. Lieberman (Eds.), *To Improve the Academy: Resources for Faculty, Instructional, and Organizational Development* (Vol. 17, pp. 103–122). Stillwater, OK: New Forums Press.

Gronlund, N.E., Linn, R.L. (1990). *Measurement and Evaluation in Teaching*. 6th Editon. New York: Macmillan Publishing Company.

Lebrun, J.L. (2010). *When the Scientist Presents*. World Scientific Publication.

McMillan, J.H. (2001). *Classroom Assessment: Principles and Practice for Effective Instruction*. Boston, MA: Allyn and Bacon.

Svinicki, M., McKeachie, W.J. (2011). *McKeachie's Teaching Tips*. Belmont, CA: Cengage Learning.

Thorndike, R.M. (1997). *Measurement and Evaluation in Psychology and Education*. Upper Saddle River, NJ: Prentice Hall.

chapter eight

Motivation

All men's souls are immortal, but the souls of the
righteous are immortal and divine.

—Socrates (470–399 BC)

8.1 Introduction

This chapter provides a variety of motivational tools for young investigators. These tools are advice, quotes, and even selected passages from short biographies such as obituaries, from great scientists demonstrating how they accomplished such greatness. They also provide with invaluable information on these scientists' general characteristics. Such information can guide young investigators in shaping their own character.

In general, I would like to mention that you will always need motivation, as there will be many obstacles in your path. However, remember that without these obstacles, the trip is not really worth it. Actually, pray for big obstacles, so you can enjoy the view from the top even more. If you go against conventional wisdom in your research, or if you will challenge the status quo in your environment, you will face tremendous adversity. I did both, and it was very difficult. But, I would rather walk on the edge, than live an ordinary life. The difference between being called a lunatic or a pioneer is really small. Personally, I take both. I really don't mind! However, one thing was certain during my personal trip. I always found refuge in the biographies and the sayings of great scientists who have walked, and are still walking, this planet.

8.2 Obituaries

You can learn a lot about excellent scientists by reading their obituaries. I like to read obituaries because they present you with inspiring facts about the individual's life. It can be very uplifting. I have listed below selected passages from several such obituaries.

8.2.1   Antoinette M. Gentile (1936–2016)

Dr. Gentile's obituary was published in the *Journal of Motor Behavior* in 2016 (Gordon et al., 2016). She was a pioneer in movement science and neuromotor research. From this obituary, I would like to mention the following passage:

> In 2009 she received the Teachers College Medal for Distinguished Service to Education. Upon receiving the Medal at the Convocation Ceremony, she provided the newly minted doctoral students hard-earned advice: "Hold fast to the questions and issues about which you are passionate."

Dr. Gentile went against conventional wisdom in her field. Her motor learning model of skill acquisition received tremendous negative criticism and resistance from colleagues, therapists, and practitioners. However, she persevered, as she believed strongly in her theory, which led to a completely new way of delivering therapy and skill training. True strength is to stand by your beliefs and discoveries.

> Ann's career required more than overcoming entrenched scientific views. In 1976, she was the first woman to be promoted to Full Professor in Teachers College's Division of Instruction. To overcome the biases of the peer review process, which favored men, Gentile also avoided using her first name, submitting and publishing papers as "A.M. Gentile." She liked to tell the story of how she was once invited to an international neuroscience conference, and had put "A.M. Gentile" next to her title for the program. She was at the opening reception when a scholar saw Gentile on her name tag and said how he very much looked forward to meeting her eminent husband, A.M. Gentile.

Dr. Gentile managed to complete two PhDs, in Physical Education and Neuropsychology, and her research work was groundbreaking. As the first female Full Professor at Teachers College, Columbia University, she faced considerable gender bias. She found her way through this adversity and she did not give up. She became a pioneer in her field and opened scientific avenues, not only for her, but for many other females.

8.2.2 Anne McLaren (1927–2007)

Dr. McLaren's obituary was published in *Science* in 2007 (Rossant & Hogan, 2007). She was a leading figure in developmental biology research. From her obituary, I would like to mention the following passages:

> She was always ready to welcome visitors, give advice, and discuss scientific matters. You were subjected to tough questioning, but in a way that led to more rigorous experiments and deeper in-sight. As many will testify, Anne was also extremely supportive of scientists struggling to work outside the main-stream or with few resources.
>
> She believed that scientists have an ethical duty to explain their research and its possible implications for society.
>
> How did she manage all this – to be an outstanding scientist, public educator and policy advisor, role model and mentor, as well as a highly involved mother and grandmother? We can only offer some clues from our experiences. She had no personal ego invested in her activities, but a strong sense of social responsibility and desire to see others succeed. Anne relished all kinds of social interactions and could party long after her younger colleagues had faded. She loved young people, and they responded in kind. And she truly did not suffer from jet lag. Anne traveled the world with one small rucksack and never seemed fatigued. She also knew how to balance family and work and to be successful at both.

From these passages, we learn a great deal about this tremendous scientist. Specifically, we learn to help other scientists who are not as fortunate as we are, to communicate our science to society, to be disciplined in our strong inference challenging others to think critically regarding their experiments, and most importantly, to properly manage our time. However, my favorite sentence is the one regarding her ego. I ask my students when they join me to give a name to their garbage can. I ask them to call it "Ego" because this is exactly where their ego belongs! Science is about giving to others, your students, society, everyone around you. Scientists should be humble and kind.

8.2.3   James F. Crow (1916–2012)

Dr. Crow's obituary was published in *Science* in 2012 (Dove & Susman, 2012). He was a prominent population geneticist whose career spanned from the modern synthesis to the genomic era. From his obituary, I would like to mention the following passages:

> Crow considered his students to be his legacy. The lecture notes for Jim's General Genetics course were so lucid and up-to date that students preferred "Crow's Notes" to their textbooks.
>
> According to Chief Justice Shirley Abrahamson of the Wisconsin Supreme Court, "his ability to teach, to listen, and to think 'outside the box' made him a respected leader."
>
> Many were perplexed that Jim could be so productive yet was so recklessly generous with his time. His daughter Cathy has explained that Jim never allowed himself to get hung up on trivia. "He was hard-working and careful, but he was not a perfectionist."
>
> Jan Klein, formerly of the Max-Planck-Institut für Biologie in Tübingen, Germany, has said that "Jim will remain as perhaps the last of a generation of gentleman-scientists 'gentleman' in the sense of a courteous, gracious man with a strong sense of honor and a strong respect for the past."

What a wonderful example of a scientist who was dedicated to his research but also to his teaching! My favorite characteristics of this legendary scientist are that he was able to think outside the box, to work hard and be meticulous while avoiding trivia, and doing all this by being a true gentleman. How can you not be inspired to emulate this individual in your life?

8.2.4   John Bennett Fenn (1917–2010)

Dr. Fenn's obituary was published in *Science* in 2011 (Muddiman, 2011). He was an analytical chemist who was awarded the 2002 Nobel Prize in Chemistry. From his obituary, I would like to mention the following passages:

> … including the importance of a strong work ethic, being open-minded in life and in science, understanding and accepting other people's struggles, and being an inspirational educator.

Clearly, John's path to the prize was serpentine and never could have been predicted by anyone, including him. He did not calculate his path to an extraordinary scientific career, but genuinely pursued ideas that were stimulating and of substantial practical value.

John was a generous and caring man with a strong sense of humility, who frequently went out of his way to make people feel comfortable. I was his colleague at VCU and remember that he would frequently say, "I learn more from my students than they will ever learn from me," a true statement from a modest man of outstanding character and vision.

Dr. Fenn's life teaches all kind of important lessons like to be humble and modest, to inspire our students and be generous with the time you dedicate to them, and to pursue ideas that are exciting but also practical (i.e. beneficial to society). These are such wonderful lessons by which to live our scientific lives.

8.2.5   Peter D. Eimas (1934–2005)

Dr. Eimas's obituary was published in *Infancy* in 2006 (Quinn & Nygaard, 2006). He was a psychologist and cognitive scientist. From his five-page-long obituary, I would like to mention the following passages:

This work would ultimately revolutionize the way that cognitive science viewed infant cognition.

and

This research was theoretically significant because of the challenge it posed to traditional learning accounts and more recent "theory-base" explanations of early concept formation.

Many great scientists have faced extreme challenges early in their career. Being a pioneer is very difficult but can also be immensely rewarding.

As a mentor of graduate students, Peter was the master. He would push one to read broadly and deeply, and with historical perspective. Excited by ideas, he emphasized keeping the big-picture questions that drive the field always in one's sights, and not losing oneself amidst the forest of parametric variation that might yield good science, but that might not, as Peter liked to put it, "tell us what we need to know." His favorite question at the end of first year graduate student talks was "What does this have to do with anything? How is this relevant?" That question became known in the folklore of Brown Psychology graduate students as the Eimas question, and one better be prepared to answer it.

It is a trademark of great scientists to cultivate the knowledge of their students in both the breadth and the depth of their discipline. My mentor, Dr. Barry T. Bates, was exactly like that. He would push me to read continuously, and in large amounts, in order to establish a solid foundation and strong understanding of the problems that existed in biomechanics. Then, when the "field" was ready, he would start "sowing." That is, he would bring everything together to develop my strong inference and my appreciation of important and most relevant questions.

In the lab, Peter left the methodological details and technological nuances for you to determine, but he was right there with you conceptually. And he taught us how to write papers! A chronic rewriter of his students' and collaborators' work as well as his own, one could usually count on Peter's feedback to start with something like "This is a good first draft, but like all first drafts it needs work." It went on from there. Writing a results section for Peter could be a little nerve-wracking. Peter's credo: Start with the tables and figures. Then run the analyses, broadest and biggest come first, more specific ones follow later.

This is very similar to what we read above, in the obituary of Dr. Crow, and we learned in the first chapter of this book. The focus should be on strong inference. Furthermore, Dr. Eimas' approach in writing papers is similar with what was mentioned in chapter four. It is fundamental to first understand the data thoroughly and then move onto the statistics and the detailed writing. There is not a better way to do so than to represent graphically what the data are revealing.

Peter practiced what he preached. On most mornings, he was the first one in the office, consistently arriving before 8:00 am. By the time you got to the lab, his office door was open, the hot tea was brewing, and in the old days, one could hear those typewriter keys clanging away. Peter wrote in the mornings, and read in the afternoons, and even on

> Sunday mornings, his orange Volvo (Peter used to say "who would steal it?") was the first to appear on the street outside of either Hunter or Metcalf Labs (or Sharpe House). When you worked with Peter, you knew you would have to bring your "A" game just to keep up with him, but the rewards were immeasurable. He took seriously the job of imparting to his students the investigative skills and confidence needed to compete with the best scientists in the world.

You cannot ask others to work hard when you do not. You cannot be a leader or a mentor without surpassing your team and your mentees in effort. You have to be with them in the trenches and the first out when the whistle blows for the attack. You need to take the bullets and not them. Dr. Eimas was such a mentor as we see from this passage.

> On a personal level, Peter was kind, generous, and fatherly. He was always available for advice. Never did a letter or an e-mail go unanswered. And as the years passed, it was Peter's lab that many graduate students turned to after their initial student–mentor relationship did not work out. As long as you were willing to work, Peter was willing to take you.

Kindness, generosity, forgiveness, and ultimately love is what Dr. Eimas gave to his mentees. This is what we all need to do as well if we want to mentor students and see them to greatness. They come as your students and they leave at least as your equals.

8.2.6   There are many others...

I could continue like this with many more such obituaries. In fact, I could dedicate an entire book to them. However, my goal was more to inspire you to pay attention to them and learn from the lessons that are hidden in them. I will also mention a few more that you can seek and read to be inspired:

- Lynn Margulis (Schaechter, 2012)
- Paul F. Barbara (Rossky & Walker, 2010)
- Benoît B. Mandelbrot (Peitgen, 2010)
- Stephen Schneider (Ehrlich, 2010)
- Lewis R. Binford (Kelly, 2011)
- John D. Roberts (Whitesides, 2016)
- Peter C. Nowell (Greene & Moore, 2017)

8.3   Profiles

Similar to the obituaries, I also like to read profiles of living scientists that are published in scientific journals. We have highlighted a few such profiles in previous chapters such as Dr. Antonio Giordano in chapter seven, and Dr. Alfredo Quiñones-Hinojosa and Dr. Anthony Fauci in chapter six. Here I will list only a couple more.

8.3.1   Daniel Shechtman

A wonderful profile of Dr. Daniel Shechtman was published in *Science* in 2011 (Clery, 2011). Dr. Shechtman was awarded the 2011 Nobel Prize in Chemistry for the discovery of quasicrystals. However, the road to his Nobel Prize was not easy as we read in this profile:

> Shechtman says he was convinced on the first day, but he checked and rechecked his experiment and tried others over the next week to investigate the material further. When he finally told colleagues about his discovery, he was met with dismissal and ridicule. His claims caused such embarrassment that his boss asked him to leave the research group. But he persevered with the help of a few colleagues, and when he finally published in Physical Review Letters in November 1984, "then all hell broke loose."
>
> But double Nobelist Linus Pauling, a dominant figure among U.S. chemists who died in 1994, never accepted quasicrystals, despite Shechtman traveling to his lab in Palo Alto and giving him a personal hour long lecture.

Dr. Shechtman was a meticulous scientist who was asking unique questions, and when serendipity came along, was ready for it like another Madame Curie. However, his discovery was met with much resistance. Dr. Shechtman persevered, though, and eventually he was justified. Several wonderful messages for young investigators arise from this profile and demonstrate important characteristics of a good scientist; perseverance, meticulousness, uniqueness in terms of the questions you ask, etc.

8.3.2   Joy K. Ward

Joy K. Ward is a notable evolutionary biologist at the University of Kansas. A profile of Dr. Ward was published in *The Scientist* in 2011 (Hopkin, 2011). From her profile, I would like to mention the following passages:

> When graduate students ask me for advice, I tell them you have to do this all the way. It's not just an eight-hour-a-day job. You have to put in the time to do great research and to develop your writing and presentation skills. If you want to be a professor and make it to the top, you have to make that decision as you begin graduate school. Because to come out of graduate school as a good researcher, a good writer, and a good speaker who knows how to think – that takes total commitment.
>
> When you have a good question, don't get held back by the historical limits of your field. You need to branch out of areas that are familiar and to learn whatever new techniques you need to answer the question.
>
> One thing as a woman scientist you need to do is to get help. Get help with your housework or with whatever you need, so you have time with your kids and time for your science. Kate Freeman from Penn State gave me that advice and I will never forget it.

Dr. Ward provides some excellent advice in her profile article about commitment, asking unique questions that could confront traditional thinking, and being a female in science. In 2009, Dr. Ward was presented with the Presidential Early Career Award for Scientists and Engineers by U.S. President Barack Obama. Therefore, we completely comprehend that Dr. Ward truly stands by her recommendations!

8.3.3   *Again there are many others...*

Similar to the obituaries, I could continue like this with many more such profiles. But again, my goal was to inspire you to pay attention to them and learn from the lessons that are hidden in them. In addition, I would like to mention that biographies could also be tremendously inspiring. I have listed a few of them at the end of this chapter as suggested additional readings.

8.4   *Advices from Nobel Prize Winners*

In this section, I would like to present some *Nature*-published content from one of the annual Lindau Nobel Laureate Meetings during which Nobel Prize winners share their experience and advice with young scientists (Nature Outlook Medical Research Masterclass, 2011). I have included below their advice in the form of vignettes followed by some personal comments.

VIGNETTE 8.1   Aaron Ciechanover
(Nobel Prize in Chemistry 2004)

"Choose a good mentor who asks original questions. Be patient, do not give up: work hard and persevere. Be passionate and excited about what you are doing: think of your scientific profession as if it were your hobby. Luck is important too, but remember, very often luck is not blind: it hits those who are ready."

In Vignette 8.1, Dr. Ciechanover suggests that the selection of your mentor should be based on the type of questions he/she is asking; original and unique questions that are based on excellent strong inference and challenge your thought processes. Dr. Ciechanover also suggests that being a scientist should be exciting. You should love your profession and you should treat it as it is your hobby. Who does not want to be a Sherlock Holmes, as we mentioned in chapter one? Lastly, luck (or serendipity as I prefer) come to those who are ready, because they work hard. As I always say to my students: "you cannot outsmart anyone, but you can outwork everybody!"

VIGNETTE 8.2   Thomas Arthur Steitz
(Nobel Prize in Chemistry 2009)

"The reason it's important to have lunch with colleagues, students, postdocs, faculty, etc., is so you can talk about ideas and experiments and science. It's a great opportunity to connect with others. See what they are doing, tell them what you're doing. I picked this up from my years at the Laboratory of Molecular Biology in Cambridge, UK[1]. Everybody would have coffee in the morning, lunch and tea together in the afternoon. They would always gather around tables and exchange ideas. It helps to stimulate thinking, to give ideas about new experiments; or you might realize that an experiment you wanted to do is perhaps not the best idea. It goes both ways. Here (at Yale University), we often have lunch with faculty from other departments, such as geology, chemistry, or physics. Obviously, you can't talk about your experiments in as much detail with these colleagues, but I have still learned a lot of interesting things, for example, about global warming, erosion of salt marshes, and rising sea levels."

---

[1] The laboratory of Molecular Biology in Cambridge University was the place where the DNA helix was discovered.

Try to have lunch with different colleagues and discuss scientific thoughts and ideas as Dr. Steitz suggests in Vignette 8.2. When I was a PhD student, I never had lunch alone; I always met with my two fellow doctoral friends and we used to bounce ideas off each other. Even if you work in different fields, you have a sounding board and are able to reciprocate. In some ways, it is even better if they are not in your field as you can gain a new perspective or a new way of looking at a problem. In addition, you may develop a friendship. Engage with your advisor – even one with a hands-off management style. The least successful students and postdocs are the ones who are silent.

VIGNETTE 8.3   Torsten Wiesel (Nobel Prize in Physiology 1981)

"The best way for the brain to work is to be exposed to different things… I see colleagues who work very hard, doing all the trivial work, but their lives miss some quality of joy."

If we read more about Dr. Wiesel, we will find that his life-long interest in art was his inspiration. He liked to mix things up a bit in his life, and his art gave him joy (Vignette 8.3). This is also important, as it allows you to masticate ideas. Many times, we produce important results and read a lot of papers, but we don't take a break so that we can truly digest the material and see the bigger picture. Creativity many times will hit you when you take a break.

VIGNETTE 8.4   Ada Etil Yonath (Nobel Prize in Chemistry 2009)

"I remember on one occasion, I made a little mistake – really just a typo. My supervisor was annoyed and questioned me about it. I apologized for it, said it was a minor error and explained that I had a lot of deadlines. He looked at me and said: "You want to stay in science? Then all your life you will be going from deadline to deadline." He was right.

Be curious – that is most important. Take passion. Be ready to sometimes experience difficulties, but enjoy what you are doing. In other words: be tough, and love your work."

Dr. Yonath is yet another great scientist who speaks about passion and love for research in Vignette 8.4. As for curiosity, well that is exactly why we are in science. She also speaks of being questioned about a single typo by her supervisor, which seems to me was a lesson in being meticulous, a trademark of great scientists. However, her supervisor also took the opportunity to mention to her that science does not stop, as it always providing you with the thrill of continuous deadlines!

VIGNETTE 8.5   Jean-Marie Lehn
(Nobel Prize in Chemistry 1987)

"Getting published is just one outcome, and not the major one. The journal in which you publish is not so important (sorry *Nature* and *Science*). What is important is that good work is recognized. It might take longer if it is published in a more obscure journal, but it still counts as being published. I can cite a number of papers that led to great discoveries but which were published in second-, third-, or fourth-rate journals. My motivation was simply that I was interested in science and research and in gaining new knowledge. All of the sciences are exciting. The great frustration is that one cannot do everything. You have to be selective to have an impact. Everybody has a given amount of energy, if you apply it on a small area you have a big impact. Too broad and the impact will be weaker."

We have a tremendous amount of excellent advice in Vignette 8.5 from Dr. Lehn. First of all: publish. Persevere and publish, even in lower impact factor journals. Aim high but widen your vision. We also see that motivation and curiosity are brought up again. Dr. Lehn also talks about channeling your energy. To achieve impactful findings in science, you must focus on a specific topic within a specific field, and that will be your niche.

VIGNETTE 8.6   Harald zur Hausen
(Nobel Prize in Physiology 2008)

"I wasn't getting much advice from my supervisor. I would go to him with crazy ideas, and he would say, "sounds interesting, why don't you try it out?" I hated it at the time because I felt like I wasn't being trained. In retrospect, however, it was a very good, creative period. I worked on a lot of nonsense, but I was able to make my own mistakes. In addition, I had the freedom to look into a lot of different areas. In turn, I tried to give my students a bit more freedom and to encourage them to develop their own ideas."

I personally use the same method with my students. My mentor was also like this. Thus, I try to provide the freedom for exploration of new ideas. Dr. Hausen, in Vignette 8.6, stresses that the lessons that you learn from your mistakes could be invaluable, and that many times, freedom leads to creativity.

VIGNETTE 8.7   Ferid Murad (Nobel Prize in Physiology 1998)

"Research is not doing what has been done before – that's confirmation. Research is doing something that's never been done before – that's creativity."

Dr. Murad advises us in Vignette 8.7 to explore new ideas and be creative. This is certainly something that will enhance our excitement about science. However, new ideas require the development of your strong inference as I have mentioned numerous times in this book.

8.5   Advices from Dr. James L. Van Etten

A few years ago, I had the pleasure of spending some time with Dr. Van Etten who is the William Allington Distinguished Professor of Plant Pathology at the University of Nebraska at Lincoln. Dr. Van Etten's numerous contributions earned him induction to the National Academy of Sciences in 2003. After more than 50 years managing his laboratory, and at the age of 81 today, Dr. Van Etten's passion for research hasn't waned. He graciously gave me several hours of his time and shared with me the following advices for young investigators.

- Talk to colleagues – Locally, nationally, internationally. You never know when someone might come up with an amazing idea.
- Be willing to take chances on an idea. You need to be willing to fail.
- Always look for interesting and unique twists on the subject you are working on.
- Publishing is very important. Try to publish in high profile journals if you can.
- Try to recruit good graduate students and postdocs to work with you. I expect them to think like scientists from the very beginning. I do not hold their hands.
- Stay off university committees!
- Work hard. I still work every day from 8:15 AM to 6:00 PM.

8.6   *The characteristics of a great scientist*

From my personal experiences, the following five characteristics are what I consider as those most important for becoming a great scientist.

1. *Be open-minded.* You must be open-minded in academia if you are to be successful. Unfortunately, as you move up the ladder in academia, your ego will also get larger and that will affect your open-mindedness. To maintain open-mindedness alongside your titles and awards, you must maintain your humility and humbleness.
2. *Be knowledgeable in a specific subject.* You must become extremely knowledgeable in your specific field. However, never stop reading scientific articles. If you are too busy, at least read the title and the abstract of every new paper that is published in your area and is generated by your automatic searches. I find time to read these articles before I go to bed, when waiting at the airport, during my flights, everywhere I can.
3. *Have intellectual curiosity and be meticulous.* If you are not curious, you will not go that extra mile. My whole dissertation topic arose because I observed something that was not mentioned in the literature. I was also meticulous, and I was able to discover it.
4. *Persevere.* Remember there is an 80% rejection rate in many journals and a single digit percentile acceptance rate at the National Institutes of Health (NIH) for many funding mechanisms.
5. *Be honest.* Scientists never judge the morality of a fact, that is, whether it's bad or good. Maintain objectivity, caution, and skepticism.

8.6   *Hints for success in science*

I close this chapter and this book with my hints for success in science. Again, these are mostly based on my own personal experiences and what I have observed or read over the years.

1. *Attend high-caliber universities.* I studied at the University of Oregon, and I was mentored by giants. I attribute a lot of my success to attending that school, which at that time, was one of the top three schools in my field.
2. *Carefully choose your research topics.* Identify a niche (see chapter one), a topic you enjoy. Also, make sure it is a *fundable* line of research. When we hire new professors in our Department, we ensure that candidates have a fundable line of research. If they perform research in topics that will never be funded from the NIH or any other governmental institution, then they have absolutely no chance of being hired by our department.

3. *Keep your research program clear and well defined.* There must be a common thread through the work that you are doing. Your work should also radiate strong inference. For example, if a student came to me saying that wanted to pursue research with me in the biomechanics of pole-vaulting, then I would say that I'm not interested. This is because it does not fit in with my research agenda. I would also be doing a disservice to the student by trying to mentor someone on a subject in which I do not have the slightest interest. I would also be doing myself a disservice, as I would not be maintaining a clear, well-defined agenda for my research work. You could have a parallel research agenda on a different topic (and this can be very beneficial – see below), but you must ensure that you have the time to perform both. Whatever you pursue, use *strong inference* and build a logical tree.

4. *Expect setbacks and be resilient.* You must expect: your grants and your manuscripts to be rejected, non-significant results, people stealing your ideas, running out of space in your lab, administrators that do not support your research, lack of funds to support your employees or to purchase the equipment you need, lack of specific expertise in collaborators where you are located, lack of patients to recruit, and so on. That is why you must be resilient. I have faced all of them!

5. *Be ready to change research topics if the likelihood of success has clearly faded.* This is exactly what happened to me. I was working initially on determining mechanisms for running injuries. I found the topic very interesting, and it was potentially fundable if I were to direct it towards osteoarthritis. However, I was not able to steer it effectively, as my grants weren't getting funded and my papers were slow to be published. I also felt that I wasn't really helping people that have serious clinical problems with my work. I decided to transition into the topic of human movement variability. This was the parallel logical tree (see chapter one) that I was working on and it was a wonderful decision.

6. *Embrace serendipity and take advantage of it quickly.* Serendipity is the gift of finding valuable things not sought for. Perhaps the most famous serendipitous moment of all is the discovery of penicillin. In 1928, Dr. Alexander Fleming took vacation and a break from his lab work investigating staphylococci. When he returned from his vacation, he found that one Petri dish had been left open, and a blue-green mold had formed. This fungus had destroyed all surrounding bacteria in the culture. The mold contained a powerful antibiotic, penicillin, that could destroy harmful bacteria without having a toxic effect on the human body. However, such moments do not happen only with Fleming or other such giants of science. It can happen to any one of you. It happened to me. I remember coming

upon with some results and thinking "Why do the curves look like that? Why is that feature never mentioned in the literature?" I know now. It ended up being the topic of my dissertation. You must take advantage of such a moment, as soon as it presents itself.

7. *Put priority on publishing your research results.* Remember that if you do not publish your research results, then THEY DO NOT EXIST. You are not contributing to science or doing yourself justice. Also, if you do not publish that work, someone else will.

8. *Find supportive mentors and avoid or leave those who are not supportive.* This has been mentioned multiple times. A non-supportive mentor is a mentor who never has time. Emails go unanswered, you don't receive feedback on papers for months, feedback is vague and unconstructive, and the list goes on.

9. *Become versed in the politics of science.* Science will always be surrounded and influenced by politics – this may be at a field-specific level, a national level, or a global level. The business meeting of your main society is a great place to learn about the things that govern how your field is progressing and its future. As a Biomechanist, the American Society of Biomechanics is my main society. At the annual meeting, I make a priority of attending the society's business meeting. Usually few attend these business meetings, but this is where all the main decisions take place. These meetings are also a great opportunity to meet important and influential scientists. I was chosen as a representative of the society and a member of the editorial board of the *Journal of Biomechanics* through attending these specific meetings. Be involved in your society. Be the student representative of your society. Be on the executive board. Many societies have a mentorship program that allows students to connect with an established scientist – take advantage of it! You can also diversify your portfolio by joining other societies. On a more national or global level, know how the political climate affects funding. Read the news. Read *Science* and *Nature*.

10. *Aim at achieving high visibility in your field.* You achieve visibility through your publications. Try to publish in high impact journals first, if possible. Aim for journals in which you want your name to be seen. To broaden your outreach, you could also try to publish in journals that are more general, or outside your field. Attend and present at conferences, dress nicely and *talk to people using your 1-min speech*. Ask scientists you respect to provide feedback on your poster or oral presentation. Utilize social media and communicate your research to everybody who is willing to listen.

11. *Work hard and do the best you can!* You cannot outsmart anyone, but you can outwork everybody!

References

Clery, D. (2011). Once-ridiculed discovery redefined the term crystal. *Science,* 334(6053), 165.

Dove, W., Susman, M. (2012). James F. Crow (1916–2012). *Science,* 335(6070), 812.

Ehrlich, P.R. (2010). Stephen Schneider (1945–2010). *Science,* 329, 776.

Gordon, A.M., Quinn, L., Kaminski, T.R., Magill, R.A. (2016). In Memoriam: Antoinette M. Gentile (1936–2016). *Journal of Motor Behavior,* 48(6), 479–481.

Greene, M.I., Moore, J.S. (2017). Peter C. Nowell (1928–2016). *Science,* 355(6328), 913.

Hopkin, K. (2011). Harvesting Ideas. *The Scientist,* 4, 50–52.

Kelly, R.L. (2011). Lewis R. Binford (1931–2011). *Science,* 332(6032), 928.

Muddiman, D.C. (2011). John Bennett Fenn (1917–2010). *Science,* 331, 160.

Grayson, M. (2011). Nature Outlook Medical Research Masterclass. *Nature,* 478(7368), S1–S20.

Peitgen, H.O. (2010). Benoît B. Mandelbrot (1924–2010). *Science,* 330(6006), 926.

Quinn, P.C., Nygaard, L.C. (2006). In Memoriam: Peter D. Eimas (1934–2005). *Infancy,* 9(2), 125–129.

Rossant, J., Hogan, B. (2007). Anne McLaren (1927–2007). *Science,* 317(5838), 609–609.

Rossky, P.J., Walker, G.C. (2010). Paul F. Barbara (1953–2010). *Science,* 330(6008), 1191.

Schaechter, M. (2012). Lynn Margulis (1938–2011). *Science,* 335(6066), 302.

Whitesides, G. (2016). John D. Roberts (1918–2016). *Science,* 354(6318), 1382.

Selected Additional Readings

Bell, E.T. (1937). *Men of Mathematics.* New York: Simon & Schuster Inc.

Bishop, J.M. (2003). *How to Win the Nobel Prize.* Boston: Harvard University Press.

Kanigel, R. (1993). *Apprentice to Genius.* Baltimore: Johns Hopkins University Press.

Mandelbrot, B.B. (2012). *The Fractalist.* New York: Vintage Books.

Quinones-Hinojosa, A. (2011). *Becoming Dr. Q.* Los Angeles: University of California Press.

Watson, J.D. (2007). *Lessons from a Life in Science.* New York: Vintage Books.

Index

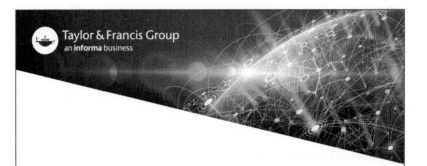